THE SECRET OF UNIVERSES

POCKET EDITION

Published from
Mardukite Borsippa HQ, San Luis Valley, Colorado
Mardukite Academy & Systemology Society
for spiritual or philosophical purposes only

THE SECRET OF UNIVERSES

Systemology
Advanced Training Course
Manual #1

As presented by Joshua Free
to the Systemology Society

© 2024, JOSHUA FREE

ISBN : 978-1-961509-47-4

This manual is restricted to students on
The Systemology Advanced Training Course
that have already completed the
"Pathway to Ascension" Professional Course

Full use of this manual may also require:
"Systemology Biofeedback" and
"Systemology Procedures"

<u>Advanced Manuals should be studied in the
sequential order in which they are numbered.</u>

First Edition Pocket Paperback — *February 2024*

mardukite.com

The Keys to the Kingdom
are Yours for the Taking!

The official Mardukite Systemology "Advanced Training Course" is now available in print for the first time.

Those Seekers that have completed the "Pathway to Ascension" Systemology Professional Course can now access the upper-level teachings of our tradition.

This book is not for everyone...
This is the first manual for Level-7.

Never before has Joshua Free presented this material outside the confines of the Mardukite NexGen Systemology Society.

Learn how to expertly apply our spiritual technology toward reaching higher levels of Awareness and Beingness than ever before thought possible for humanity.

Each of the "Keys to the Kingdom" Advanced Training Course Manuals will further a Seekers reach on the Pathway leading out of this Universe.

<u>The Pathway to Ascension</u>
Professional Course Lesson Booklet Series

#1 – *Increasing Awareness (Level-0)*
#2 – *Thought & Emotion (Level-0)*
#3 – *Clear Communication (Level-0)*
#4 – *Handling Humanity (Level-1)*
#5 – *Free Your Spirit (Level-2)*
#6 – *Escaping Spirit-Traps (Level-2)*
#7 – *Eliminating Barriers (Level-3)*
#8 – *Conquest of Illusion (Level-3)*
#9 – *Confronting the Past (Level-4)*
#10 – *Lifting the Veils (Level-4)*
#11 – *Spiritual Implants (Level-5)*
#12 – *Games and Universes (Level-5)*
#13 – *Spiritual Energy (Level-6)*
#14 – *Spiritual Machinery (Level-6)*
#15 – *The Arcs of Infinity (Level-6)*
#16 – *Alpha Thought (Level-6)*

<u>Keys to the Kingdom</u>
Advanced Training Course Manuals

#1 – *The Secret of Universes (Level-7)*
#2 – *Games, Goals & Purposes (Level-7)*
#3 – *The Jewel of Knowledge (Level-7)*
#4 – *Implanted Universes (Level-7)*

Advanced Training Supplemental Booklets
#1 – *Systemology Biofeedback*
#2 – *Systemology Procedures*

TABLET OF CONTENTS

INTRODUCTION TO THE MANUAL

A.T. MANUAL #1:
THE SECRET OF UNIVERSES

APPENDIX

INTRODUCTION TO
THE MANUAL

This manual is restricted to students on
The Systemology Advanced Training Course
that have already completed the
"Pathway to Ascension" Professional Course

Full use of this manual may also require:
"Systemology Biofeedback" and
"Systemology Procedures"

THE SYSTEMOLOGY
ADVANCED TRAINING COURSE
MANUAL SERIES

Mardukite Systemology is a new evolution in Human understanding about the "systems" governing *Life, Reality*, the *Universe* and all *Existences*. It is also a *Spiritual Path* used to transcend the Human experience and reach *"Ascension."*

This is an *Advanced Training* (*AT*) course manual detailing *upper-levels* of our spiritual philosophy. It is intended to assist *advancing* a *Seeker's* personal progress toward the *upper-most levels* of the *Pathway*.

This manual follows after our *Professional Course* series of lessons—available as individual booklets, or collected in two volumes titled *"The Pathway to Ascension"* The *Professional Course* follows after material given in the *Basic Course* booklets, or *"Fundamentals of Systemology"* volume.

The systematic methodology that we use to assist an individual to increase their *"Actualized Awareness"* (and reach gradually higher toward their *"Spiritual Ascension"*) is referred to as *"The Pathway"* — and that individual is called a *"Seeker."*

To receive the greatest benefit from this manual: it is expected that a *Seeker* will already be familiar with the fundamental concepts and terminology (previously relayed in the *Basic Course* and *Professional Course* lessons) of our *applied philosophy.*

As a *Seeker* increases their *Awareness* in this lifetime, their spiritual *"Knowingness"* also increases—which is to say their *certainty* on *Life*, on this and other *Universes*, and on *realizing Self* as an unlimited "spiritual being" *having* an enforced restrictive "human experience." A *Seeker* also *knowingly* increases their command and control of the "human experience." And this is a part of what is meant by *"Actualized Awareness."*

CHARTING FLIGHTS ON THE PATHWAY

Although there is a systematic structure to *fragmentation,* the personal journey experienced along the *Pathway* will be different for each *Seeker.* For example, certain areas will seem more *"turbulent"* or difficult for one *Seeker* than another. We tend to say that these areas have more *"charge"* on them—or that they are more *"heavily charged."* It is best to handle such areas when you are already feeling "good" and not in a situation (or condition) where that specific area is consistently being *"triggered"* or *"restimulated."*

As an applied philosophy, *Systemology* "theory" can be easily utilized in the "laboratory" of the "world-at-large" in everyday life. This is implied within the basic instruction of each lesson. Unlike other "sciences" that conduct experiments by making a change to some "objective variable" *out there* and waiting to see an effect, our focus is the individual (or *Observer*) themselves, and how *they* affect the "*Reality*" perceived.

Our philosophy is applied by using specific exercises and systematic techniques. These "*processes*" provide the most stable personal gain (and *realizations*) for each area; but only when actually applied with a *Seeker's* full "*presence*" and *Awareness*. Hundreds of such *processes* may be found in the "*Pathway to Ascension*" (*Professional Course*) material.

Applying a technique is called "*running a process.*" *Processes* are designed with very simple instructions or "*command-lines.*" To *run* a *processing command-line*, a *Seeker* may be assisted by the communication of that *line* from a "*Co-Pilot*" (as in "*Traditional Piloting*"). But even then, a *Seeker* must still personally "input" the *command* as *Self.* For this reason—and quite thankfully—*Solo-Processing* is possible.

TAKING FLIGHT ON THE PATHWAY

Processing Techniques are intended to treat the *Spiritual Being* or *Alpha-Spirit*; the individual themselves. The *"command-lines"* are *directed to* the individual themselves— not some *mental machinery* of theirs, and not even a *Biofeedback* metering device.

Systematic Processing is applied by the *Alpha-Spirit*—who then *Self-directs* command of their "Mind-System" or "body" (*genetic-vehicle*), both of which are "constructs" that the *Alpha-Spirit* (*Self*, or the "I-AM" *Awareness unit*) operates, but neither of which is actually *Self*. *Fragmentation* causes *Humans* to falsely identify *Self as* the "*Mind*" or even a "*Body.*"

Some *processes* can be treated quite lightly at first; others may require a bit of working at in order to get *"running"* well. It is important to set aside a period of time when you can be dedicated to your studies and *processing*. This period of time is referred to as a *"processing session."* When a *process* does start *running* well, it is important to be able to complete it to a satisfactory *"end-point."*

Processing allows us to be able to *actually* "look" at *things* and even determine the *considerations* we have made—or attitudes we have decided—about *Reality* as a result of those experiences.

It doesn't do us much good to simply "glance"—or to *restimulate* something uncomfortable and then quickly *withdraw* from it once again, leaving more of our *attention* yet again behind and held fixedly on it.

Generally speaking, a *Seeker* continues to *run* a *process* so long as something is "happening"—which is to say, the *process* is still producing a change. Usually this is evident by the type of "answers" that a *command-line* prompts a *Seeker* to originate from the database of their own *Mind-System*.

Processing Command-Lines ("PCL") are not "magic words"; they do not "do" anything on their own. They systematically assist a *Seeker* to direct their own attention toward increasing *Awareness*.

A *Seeker* may also cease to generate new "data" from a *process* without reaching an "ultimate" realization as an "end-point." It is possible that additional "layers" (or even other "areas") require handling before anything "deeper" is accessible. If this is the case, end the *process*. But, if a *Seeker* is *withdrawing* from something uncomfortable that was incited or stirred up, then a *process* is *run* until they feel "good" about it.

One of the benefits to *Flying-Solo* on the *Pathway* is that the *processing* is entirely *Self-determined*. This naturally provides a

17

certain built-in "safety" for a practitioner. Anything you *restimulate* by *Self-determinism* is *your thing*. It is not triggered or incited by some external "*other-determined*" influences (or other "source-points") that make you an *effect*. It can be more easily handled in *processing*—or you can simply let things "cool down" and come back to it again in another *session*.

While it may seem "mysterious" to beginners, a *Seeker* gets a sense for knowing how long to *run* a *process* only with practice. Once you have spent some time actually applying material from "*The Pathway to Ascension*" *Professional Course*, there are many aspects of it that become "second nature" because they are, in fact, a part of our true original native nature. All we have done in *Systemology* is "*reverse engineer*" the routes of *creation* and *consideration* that are already *our own*.

Advanced Manuals should be studied in the sequential order in which they are numbered.

A.T. MANUAL #1
THE SECRET OF
UNIVRESES

> "MANY YEARS AGO, I REALIZED THAT 'THE WAY OUT' WOULD SYSTEMATICALLY RESEMBLE THE ROUTES BY WHICH WE ORIGINALLY DESCENDED."
>
> —*Joshua Free*
> *Backtrack Lectures*

THE SECRET DOCTRINE

Upon *"initiation"* to *Systemology Level-7*, a *Seeker* is introduced to our *"Secret Doctrine."* This is *not* religious dogma; it does not even require *belief* or *faith*. It is, however, what our *Pathway* is structured after —including the *levels* that have delivered a *Seeker* to this point. It is *"secret"* only for the fact that an individual will not likely *confront* its *reality*, or even *understand* it, prior to reaching this advanced point on the *Pathway*.

"The Secret Of Universes" manuscript provides additional *context* to the information a *Seeker* has already explored on the *"Pathway to Ascension"* *Professional Course*; because elements of it directly appeared in those course materials. Those details already given about certain areas will not be repeated here. Details provided in later materials of the *Keys to the Kingdom*

Advanced Training Course will not be included here.

This is a very *bold* narrative. It is not meant to be discouraging; but informative. At the very least we must be able to *confront* where we have been—and how we got to where we are—if we hope to ever retrace our steps and find our way back out again.

What *is* included here is a general outline —the basic *systematic structure*—of our *Cosmic Spiritual History*; the most important and necessary parts for broadly understanding the *"bigger picture."* To elaborate further would *evoke* individual perspectives, cultural interpretations, or differing languages used to assign proper names. Any such treatments and/or speculations are outside the purpose of this manuscript.

Only small parts of this *"big picture"* have been *glimpsed* before—in shreds and tears. This is due to imperfect *fragmented communications* by traditions that became so fixed upon "kabbalistic symbols" and "correspondence charts" that any truer meaning of the *Secret Doctrine* was long forgotten. Our *communication* of it, in *Systemology*, will be much more direct—and *systematic*.

The subject of *Universes* is introduced directly in *Professional Course (PC) Lesson-12*. Other *upper-level* concepts—*Spiritual Implants* and *Spiritual Machinery*, *&tc.*—will also be mentioned in this narrative. A *Seeker* is encouraged to refer to appropriate materials when certain subjects emerge that require more clarity.

This *lore* remains an "esoteric secret"—even when published in plain sight—because it is rarely understood properly. The average person is going to have little *reality* on this material at all. Meanwhile, a *Seeker* that has completed the "*Pathway to Ascension*" *Professional Course* might look at it and say, *"well, of course, how could it be any other way?"* In either case, no *enforcement* is suggested about "believing" anything.

Unlike other *Systemology* lessons and booklets, this manuscript does not include *processing* instructions or exercises. It does, however, include a lot of information and *points to "spot"* in later *Advanced Training (AT) Course* materials. Any *reactivity* or *turbulence* encountered while reading this should be noted, then handled with techniques from the *PC* material (or as described in the *"Systemology Procedures" AT Supplement*). Later *AT* course manuals will treat more specific points of this manuscript with data that is not already given.

Those *Seekers* that have not reached a basic state of *Beta-Defragmentation* yet—or are still working through *PC* material for the first time—should take care to assign specific uninterrupted time in a safe place to initially study this material. When first reading this, it is not uncommon for some individuals to go *"unconscious"* (*fall asleep*) when more information is read in one sitting/session than they are prepared to *confront* all at once. This may not even happen. But if it does: make a record of where it happened and then pick it up again from an earlier point.

A *Universe* is a *complete system* of *space-time*. This discourse is primarily concerned with those *large agreed-upon Universes* that we have all inhabited. *Universes* have become more "solid." We often refer to this as the *"Condensation of Universes."* Other *Universes* do not reflect the same *"Physical Laws"* as *this Beta-Existence.* And superior to all of these, is the *individual* as their *own Personal Universe.*

In previous *PC* lessons, an individual's *Personal Universe* and *"Home Universe"* were treated as one and the same concept and elevated to the highest position on the *Standard Model* (encompassed only by the *Infinity-of-Nothingness*). In *this* manual, we will reveal that this was a great oversimplification of the facts (which had simply seemed adequate for previous purposes).

IN THE BEGINNING...

Before *"Home Universe"*—before all *Existence*—there can only be an *Infinity-of-Nothingness.* It exists before and back of all *Space* and *Time.* It is, itself, unchanging. But within it is the infinite *Potential-of-Everythingness*; because an *infinity of creation* has descended from that *Nothing.*

The *Nothing* has the *potential* for *"thought"*—but there is *nothing* to think about until *something* is *created.* The very *first "Alpha" thought*, and *first "Alpha" creation*, are one and the same. The *process* of

Alpha-Thought, in its highest form, is the *process of creation*.

Considering the basic components of a *Universe—Space, Time, Energy* and *Matter* —only one is senior, or rather, first, above the others; only one can be considered without a reference to the others—and that is *Space*. Inherent to *Space*, is the concept of *separation*. At first, the only 'thing' *there* to separate, *was* the *Infinity-of-Nothingness*. And this *separateness* resulted in "*Alpha Spirits*."

An "*Alpha Spirit*" is essentially a *fragment* of the basic *Infinity-of-Nothingness*. By its *separateness*, it becomes a basic *individual* unit of *Spiritual Awareness* itself. It is not affected by this separation. At basic, the "*Alpha Spirit*" remains a part of the *Nothingness*, but with a potential for *infinite creation*—and the capability to *experience time*; meaning an ability to perceive conditions of *having* and *not-having* their *creations*.

Once the *Awareness Unit* is *aware* (can *conceive*) that it has *separated*, then it applies further *separations* to bring about the *creation of existence*. *Space* is the *separation* of "parts" or "particles." *Time* is the *separation* of "incidents" or "events." *Identity* then becomes necessary for the *separation* of "thought." Without *identity*, all *thought* would be "one"—and that is apparently too passive of a condition for *creation* to occur.

The *Infinity-of-Nothingness* is beyond *all considerations* of *Space-Time*; it therefore remains "*Infinity*" from our perspective of *Space-Time*. Its very nature exceeds whatever *infinite creation* is manifest; it continuously demands further *infinities of somethings* to balance its *nothingness*.

Since it is a basic part of us, we never are disconnected from, or lack, the *nothing*. Our sense of lack is always in the direction of *somethings* (that are not *nothing*), of which we will always come up short of balancing the *Nothingness* completely.

At basic, the *Spiritual Awareness Unit* is the *Total Sum of All Potential Awareness*. It simply *IS*; and it is superior (above) to its other *considerations* of *Space, Time, Energy* and *Matter*. *Matter* is a *consideration* that *something* is *there*. *Energy* is a *potential* for *something* to *happen*. As *Self-Aware* beings, *Alpha-Spirits* (*Alpha-Thought Units of Infinity*) fulfill their basic function by continuing an ongoing sequence of *infinite creation*. [Only when this *creativeness* is "blocked" or "restricted" do we become "unhappy." All lesser states are thus slightly unpleasant; but the idea of future *creations* drives us forward.]

Our separation from the *Infinity-of-Nothingness* is only a *consideration*. The *Alpha-Spirit* is still a part of the basic state; it never really "left" and thus there is no reason to "rejoin." The "*Pathway to Ascension*" or "*Return to Source*" is not a dissolving of *Identity* back into a "pool" of *Nothingness*. This is a false assumption that is easy to make. The *Infinity-of-Nothingness* is not "enlarged" or "enhanced" by that "reincorporation" and as a result, does not even allow for it.

At our highest state of co-existence with the *Nothingness*, each individual *is*, for all intents and purposes: *God*—and with a basic function: *To Create*. Although there is a certain inherent *timelessness* to this state, there is also a sequence, perceived by existing *Alpha-Spirits*, of "newer beings" coming forth from the *Infinite*. Freshly separated "beings" would then *create* "new systems" not already in *existence*.

Of course, the newest and most original *creations* and *systems* would result from "fresh beings" that could be isolated from any exposure to existing *creations* conceived by "older beings." A phenomenon began to occur where a new batch of "fresh beings" were isolated into *"pockets of infinity"* or *"wombs of creation."*

All of us here now are presently in such a *"pocket"* or *"womb."* And the entire series of *Universes* we have *created* (and inhabited) have all existed within *this "womb."* When we have completed our *progression*, we can then *exit the womb* and carry our *creations* and *systems* with us to blend with those of "older beings." And when we have exhausted every variation and combination thereof, we will then usher in the next batch of "fresh beings" who will also play their part in this dance of *infinite creation*.

Of course, initially isolating a group of *god-like* beings requires a bit of work. We are speaking of the basic state of an *Alpha-Spirit*, with the ability to *create* and *destroy Universes* on a whim. Of course, since you are initially dealing with "fresh"—"innocent"—beings, you may be able to misdirect their *attention* for awhile; but they will eventually start to notice the more elaborate *creations* of the "older beings." Something more *systematic* is necessary.

A *god-like* being can only *limit* (or *"trap"*) itself. *"False data"* and *"deception"* from others can certainly encourage this. But even so, the "older beings" cannot directly involve themselves in the *process*. The batch of "fresh beings" must be *tricked* into being in *conflict* with others in order to *create "traps."* And it is the *"traps"* we *created* for others that really ended up *trapping* ourselves.

The *systematic sequence* at play here is for the "fresh beings" to *create* their own *traps.* By sinking deeper into them, they will eventually become the *"effect"* of their own *creations*. This leads to a *"spiritual amnesia"* (reduced *Awareness* and *Knowingness*) concerning their own *Identity* and the nature of their *creations*. By forgetting (*Not-Knowing*) how the *trap* was made, a new *systemology* had to evolve to reveal the *structure* of the *trap*. And this is used to regain *control* of our *creations* and dig ourselves out of the *trap* —and *Ascend*.

As *Alpha Spirits*, we may pretend to be *older* or *higher* than others. But we are all existing now at the bottom of such a *trap*. We have reached a state where we can only *create* with *atoms* and *particles* provided to us. It's time to dig ourselves out and *exit the womb*. The "older beings" cannot intervene. The only *"way out"* is to regain our *spiritual power*—and that means regaining *control* of our *creations*. They are, after all, *our creations*.

BEFORE "HOME UNIVERSE"

We have been isolated away from "older beings" in this *womb* for a very long time.

There is only one instance of "contact" that we have ever had with *them*, one single encounter with a *creation* from them—and it occurs at the very beginning. While there have been many *"false beginnings"* (suggested by *Implants*), and many *"starts-of-time"* upon *entry-to-a-Universe*, there is only one true *first experience* —and we have all had it.

As we separated from the *Infinity-of-Nothingness*, our *attention* was directed to something so *fascinating* that it drew us in before we could think of *looking* at anything else. We call this *"The Jewel of Knowledge."* We might have expected our first experience to be incredibly simple or basic, but instead, it is perhaps the most *complex creation* we have ever beheld—because it came from "outside" and was *created* by "older beings." It *showed* us what we were supposed to do.

Complexity of *The Jewel* can only be vaguely described here. Although it was "diamond-like" in shape, it was intentionally designed with more *facets* (or *faces*) in more dimensions than we could even perceive all at once in our native state. This is what *compelled* us to *look* so closely. When *"scanning"* Incidents on the Backtrack, there are many *"false jewels"* (attached to later, more recent, *Implants*) that only imitate the *systematic structure* of *The Jewel*, but certainly not the *complexity*. [These "imitations" are what we treat at *Systemology Level-7*, as indicated in the *AT Course* manual titled: *"The Jewel Of Knowledge."*]

The Jewel of Knowledge contained many "chambers"—each of which we experienced sequentially; each of which demonstrated something interesting and useful to a "fresh being." Some of the *"knowledge"* was "correct." Some parts subtly encouraged a tendency toward *conflict* and *creating traps*.

The original *Jewel* does not communicate

using a "language." Much of it is displayed with *geometry*, which itself, lays in a *structure* for *creation*—but it never shows anything that we would consider a "*Body*." Other individuals (and groups of beings) are generally indicated by "points of light" or "nebulous clouds."

Most of the "chambers" provided simple demonstrations. For example: one of the first ones showed how to *perceive an object*. It demonstrates setting up "*viewpoints*" from various directions (or dimensions) in order to permeate or pervade the totality of what you're *looking* at. A "two-dimensional" *creation* is *perceived* in its totality only from "three" (or more) dimensions, *&tc.* Of course, *The Jewel of Knowledge* might demonstrate this with a "seven-dimensional cube." Many other "basic" *shapes* and *structures* are also used.

Some "chambers" demonstrated more *misleading data*. For example: one might depict many individuals working together in harmony to *create* pieces of an object and the idea is that things are pleasant. Then one of the beings goes against the efforts of the others and things become unpleasant. The group of beings collectively force the individual back into agreement, and the scenery is pleasant and harmonious again. It doesn't take a lot of analysis for us to see what this is intended to impress.

By the time our journey through the "chambers" is complete, we're set up with the idea that it is necessary to *control* and *trap* other *Alpha-Spirits*. There is also an impression made on us that in exchange for this *Jewel* we would have to *create* something of our own; only then would we be allowed to see other *creations* (made by the "older beings"). Of course, here we are, still working on this *ultimate creation* (apparently); and in the meantime, have dug ourselves pretty deep into it. We've forgotten we really wanted to be *outside* of it all.

After our *Jewel* experience, we were excited to begin *creating* an interesting and complex *Universe*. Of course we weren't "alone." Each *Alpha-Spirit* in this state was a *god-like* being; each one charged with remaining an *individual*, yet keeping *others* in line—and thus ensuring *conflict*. [*Implants* generally contain "*false data*" because they are structured so that we equally hold these kinds of *opposing considerations* simultaneously.]

The *Jewel* provided no requirements or specific rules for *creation*; not even a set number of dimensions to use. This actually led to the first primary *conflict* between *Alpha-Spirits*. Each of us chose, for whatever reason, a certain number of dimensions (from *one* to as many as *twelve*) to start working on. We found ourselves developing these *systems* with others that had also selected that number of dimensions.

As an *Alpha-Spirit* spent more *time* and *effort* working with a particular number of dimensions, they felt a certain attachment to the *systems* they were invested in. Those working on a lower number of dimensions started producing results more quickly than the rest. For example: complete "two-dimensional" *systems* resembled something like what we consider "board games" (like "chess") today. The "one-dimensional" *system* known as "music" or "musical notes" still remains with us in *Beta-Existence*.

Seeing how those working on "lower-dimensions" were yielding faster results, the *Alpha-Spirits* working on the "higher-dimensional" *creations* started realizing how far they still had to go to make real progress. Slowly, those working on "higher" numbers began to shift over to "lower" ones. Since the "one-" and "two-dimensional" *systems* were already being perfected, most of the shifts were to "three" through "five" (where room for new contributions still remained).

As the "three-dimensional" *systems* were nearly completed, it became obvious (to these "*Threes*") that those *Alpha-Spirits* remaining "above" to work on higher-dimensional *systems* would eventually shift to work with the "*Fours*" or "*Fives*" (and not join them as "*Threes*"). This wouldn't have been an issue except that *The Jewel* had impressed that everyone must be "in line" and *agree* upon a single *system*.

The "*Threes*" also knew they could be "outnumbered" this way; and that the "four-dimensional" *systems* could overwhelm and manipulate their own *creations*, just as operating from "three-dimensions" allows one to crumple up a "two-dimensional" *painting*, or toss sweep a *game board* off a table. For a moment, the "*Threes*"—with their nearly complete *system*—held a temporary advantage over the *"Fours."* Rather than wait to be "inevitably" subdued, the *"Threes"* attacked first; and this started the *"Reality Wars."*

Relatively speaking, the *Reality Wars* represent the *longest era* of our *Spiritual History*. When you consider the tremendous ability exercised by an *Alpha-Spirit* in this *god-like* state—essentially invulnerable to everything except the *effects* of their *own considerations* and *decisions*—it took an exceptionally long time for these beings to wear each other down to a point of making a mutually shared *reality-agreement*.

In the end, the *"Threes"* successfully laid in "mental" *barriers* that interfered with *creating* and *perceiving* higher-dimensional *systems*. They could not "block" the lower-dimensions in this wise, because they were an integral part of their own. And, of course, the *"Fours"* could not retaliate in this way, for the same reasons.

This has left us with a "three-dimensional" structure for *Universe Systems* ever since. Although they have never been as rigidly *"solid"* as we experience today, the basic visible or apparent form of "things" as being "three-dimensional objects" has been considered "normal" to us for a very long time.

During the final *conflict* of the *Reality Wars*, the *"Fours"* were successful in one particular counter-attack: *Implanting* a *compulsive desire* for *four-dimensional creations*. As an illustrative physical example: a single "four-dimensional trading card" might satisfy the desire *to collect trading cards.* But since this is not achievable in any *Beta-Existence*, the *dramatization* (or reactive behavior) is *to collect* an endless amount of "three-dimensional trading cards" in an attempt to reach the same condition (as owning *one* 4-D card).

Alpha-Spirits have experienced a strange state of affairs ever since the *Reality Wars* ended. Although we all fell in line on the "three-dimensional" nature of *apparent creation*, the "four-dimensional" component was not eliminated. We stopped being able to *perceive* it, yet we still could *react* to those *creations* and even craved them. Even our *Universe* gains its "*solidity*" by having a special kind of 4-D "*thickness*" to it. Almost as if *reality* is actually multiple layered copies all moving together.

THE ALPHA-SPIRITS

For the era of the *Reality Wars*, we are still referring to *Spiritual Beings* with practically unlimited ability *to create* and *to alter creations*. *Alpha-Spirits* were still quite capable of placing their *Beingness* (as *Awareness*) in many places simultaneously; and managing many complex functions at the same time ("remote" from one another). We were, however, inexperienced; our *understanding* was still quite limited to *considering* only the *mechanics* and *structure* of *"things"* —without any real *"significance"* or *"meaning"* attached.

As we still all occupied the "level" of *Alpha-Thought*, *our* earliest *communications* with others were pure exchanges of *"Knowingness."* You would just *"Know"* someone *intended* for you to come and *look* at their *creation*. So, you would go *look* and *intend* (or *decide*) that they would *"Know"* whether or not you liked it. Then they could *intend/decide* you to *"Know"* if they were satisfied or unsatisfied with your opinion.

The first *communications* using "abstract symbol pictures" began at the start of the *Reality Wars*. It is actually in the area of *communication* that we first became *fragmented*; and it is this area that we must treat first, at the very beginning of the *Pathway-to-Ascension* (and our corresponding *"Professional Course"* series for it). Efforts to limit *communication* began with *The Jewel of Knowledge*, to influence "fresh beings" not to attempt to *communicate* with the "outside" (or "older beings")—and also to further incite *conflicts* "inside." Individuals don't "fight" or "entrap" each other when they are maintaining *clear communication*.

Unlike other forms of *fragmentation*, these first *"communication flow-breaks"* were *Self-determined*. While the specific preferences differed between us, we each began making decisions about *"who"* or *"what"* we no longer wished to be in *communication* (*contact*) with. And this is a key to our *way out*. Since these early basic *communication barriers* were *created* by choice, then they can easily be dissolved (*defragmented*) by *deciding* to resume such *communication* again (without even having to sort out the many layers piled onto this area).

Today, a *Seeker* applies *systematic processing* to peel back many layers of *fragmentation* that have accumulated on the *foundations* of previous *Implants* and *Incidents*. But early in our existence, our problems mainly resulted from *unwillingness to communicate* and *incomplete communications*. Misunderstandings are what led to the first *upsets* and *harmful-acts* experienced by an *Alpha-Spirit*. We're not inherently *evil*; just *fragmented*.

At this early point in *existence*, an *Alpha-Spirit* is still unable to be affected by *"energy-waves"* or *"force."* Any *"implanting traps"* required more subtlety. They were *created* to hold one's *attention* by being *aesthetically* "beautiful" or "interesting"—similar to the "chambers" of *The Jewel*. Some were just "viewable." Others might allow you to totally immerse yourself in the experience within a *holograph-*

ic-like micro-verse. Although we couldn't be *"harmed,"* we were being encouraged to *"tune down"* our *spiritual abilities* the whole time.

We operated on both sides of this—being the *cause* and *effect* of the *traps*—and switched sides often. Most of it didn't affect us very much until we eventually slid into *traps* we forgot we had *created* ourselves (during a period of playing for the "other side"). [It apparently never occurred to anyone to only *create traps* that could not *entrap* their own *creator*.]

After the *Reality Wars*, a constriction to "three-dimensions" was the only *enforced reality-agreement*. There was still no single *agreed-upon Universe*. As a result of the long era of *conflict*, everyone remained in a highly "disagreeable" state. When an individual *created* something, someone might change its purpose or nature, meanwhile someone else might *create* something to render it useless, *&tc*. It was a period of one-upmanship (out-doing each other as rivals) and disrupting the *creations* of others. This only led to further *problems* and us going further *out-of-communication* with each other.

When we experienced *The Jewel of Knowledge*, we were practically omniscient and not actually "located" anywhere, except that our *attention* could be focused on something (like *The Jewel*). But, *The Jewel* also convinced the *Alpha-Spirit* that it should locate a *"mass"* or *"anchor-point"* in *spaces* it was operating from. *The Jewel* implanted *"false data"* that *Space* should be "owned," but could only belong to an *individual* that had its *"mass"* there. An intermediate period consisted of a lot of multi-verse/micro-verse *creation activity* — but nothing yet *agreed-upon* (except the *dimensions* of *form*).

An *Alpha-Spirit's consideration* of its own *Beingness* starts to "*condense*" as it begins to believe that it is in any way "located" where its *"masses"* are. Prior to the first *agreed-upon Universe*, the *Alpha-Spirit* could still "occupy" many different *viewpoints* simultaneously and remote from each other—even when it started to *consider itself* as "located." But this all changed when we realized one common area of *agreement*: we still had yet to *create* something together that compared with *The Jewel*.

So, we built our first *agreed-upon Universe* —and we "located" ourselves there as *individuals*.

This *"Agreements Universe"* was a gigantic wide-open three-dimensional *Space*. It was poorly planned. In fact, it had no real organizational structure at all, except for an *agreed-upon* set of *"definitions"*—which were also greatly flawed. The *definitions* were set up as *"dichotomies"*—*"pairs of opposites"* (*e.g.* "good"/"bad"). For whatever reason, the *"pairs"* didn't really align with each other in a way that made sense—

resulting in more *miscommunication* and *entrapment*.

A *"Shared Universe"* requires that everyone within it *share* some specific *universal parameters* or *reality-agreements*, whatever they may be. If we all operate from fully independent and separate *Space-Times*, there is no way to be in *communication* with those "outside" of that (others that are operating independently on their own set of *reality-agreements*). It makes it quite difficult to *create* and/or *play* together.

As a mundane example: if one person is operating as though today is "Wednesday," and everyone else is showing up because it's "Thursday" on their calendar, the individual is not *in-phase* with the *schedule*/*reality* of the *group*. Even in modern times, we would tend to consider those individuals as "in their own world."

The *definitions* were collected together — and we *agreed* to follow them even before we had inspected them all. We each had only participated in developing one or some of them and hadn't really seen what the others were. We all believed that everyone should have a part in *defining* the basic *reality-agreements* necessary to experience the *Shared-Universe* with each other. This led to manufacturing a *"Reality-Implant"* or *"Universe-Implant"* that didn't come from "outside" (like *The Jewel*).

To *create* and *experience* the *Agreements Universe* required an *Implant Construct*, whereby an individual would "enter in" and be subjected to *enforced agreements* for the *reality* of that *Universe*. Its design was modeled after *The Jewel*, using "facets" or "chambers" to show various "picture sequences." The imagery was quite elementary, rather like the "picture books" we use to *indoctrinate* children with today.

51

The sequences were built into a four-dimensional *construct.* Although our true four-dimensional *abilities* and *perceptions* were blocked (after the *Reality Wars*), these beings were still able to get together and layer so many copies of a three-dimensional *creation* that it extended into the fourth-dimension (to maintain its *structure*) as a *Universal "Entry-Point."* It was essentially a "portal" or "gate" *from* the *"Misaligned Zone"* (remaining from the *Reality Wars*) *into* the *Agreements Universe.*

Rather than the more elaborate *"diamond"* structure of *The Jewel of Knowledge*, this *construct* appeared as an *"inverted golden pyramid,"* which represented the "narrowing down" of *realities* into *one*. Each of the three-dimensional "pyramid chambers" composed a *"part"* or *"facet"* of the four-dimensional *"hyper-pyramid."* Each "pyramid chamber" established (or "implanted") a *reality-agreement* about one of the *"dichotomies."*

We all gathered together and dived through the *Inverted Golden Pyramid Implant* together. [On the *Backtrack*, you can "*Spot*" the sense of "*rushing to get into agreement*" that is attached to this *Incident*. Thousands of other *Alpha-Spirits* are also rushing through. You pass through the "pyramid chambers" and receive the *Universe-Implanting*.] We all emerge from it into a unified *infinite space* that is faintly golden in color, rather than "dark."

At this point of our existence, the concept of "death" (in any way) did not yet exist. At worst, we might choose to "forget" (*Not-Know*) things; or abandon one area of *Space* and go off to the other "side" of the *Universe* and continue our *creating*.

We had not yet fixed our *Beingness* "inside" or "interior to" any of our *creations*. However, there was a tendency to create "body forms" (to represent us) that mirrored the scenery of the *Implant* (rather than "pyramids" and "spheres" from our previous existence). These weren't the kind of "solid bodies" used today; they could flick in or out of existence and we weren't connected to them. If one got "zapped," you could just make another.

The *Agreements Universe* was an interesting era of fluid ever-changing *creation*; but it led to many problems. A loose structure of *reality-agreements* resulted in *conflict*—"tricking" each other; "messing up" each other's *creations, &tc*. No one could get invested into a *complex creation* —or some grandiose *aesthetic art construct* —without someone else making something "weird" (an anomaly) "pop up" in the middle of it. Everyone got pretty frustrated with these conditions. The solution was to develop a new *Universe* that could be *infinitely fractioned* in such a way that each *Alpha-Spirit* could have their own complete "*Home Universe.*"

"HOME UNIVERSE"

While we tend to treat *"Home Universe"* as *"7.0"* on our *Systemology models* and *scales*, it actually occurred midway in our *Spiritual Existence*. It is, however, at this point, that we start to keep track of *"time"*—mainly for *sequencing* conditions of *"having"* and *"not having"* and to *realize* a *"chronology"* of events. For this reason, data from here onward is easier to "contact" when handling the *Backtrack* directly. The previous events described—from *The Jewel of Knowledge* up to this *Home Universe*—are far more obscure and abstract to *conceive*.

In many ways, *Home Universe* was the "apex" of our existence. We still had amazing *creative ability* and had not yet taken on much *spiritual fragmentation*. Each individual *Alpha-Spirit* had their own *infinite space* to *create* in, which was separate from everyone else. But they were still all connected by a *"matrix"* of *higher-level Space.*

The *Home Universe Matrix* linked the individual *Home Universes* together. But this *Matrix* should not be *considered* a *Universe* full of little *spheres* inhabited by each *Alpha-Spirit.* [A later, more recent, *Implant* does suggest this imagery however.] Each *Home Universe* was literally an *infinite space.* The *Matrix* acted like an inter-dimensional "corridor" or "hallway" that simply connected them all; it expanded to encompass each *Home Universe*, giving each the appearance of a having a distant *"night sky full of stars."*

These *"stars"* were not like the *"suns"* you find in *the Physical Universe.* They were luminous *"orbs"* that served as the original *"Star-Gates"* (we encounter on the *Backtrack*). Each *Star-Gate* connected to another individual *Home Universe* (each of which contained an *infinite space*). Each

Home Universe was one's own. It did not have to follow or share any strict "physical laws" with other *Home Universes*. The only commonalities were the *"entry-points"* (maintained by the *Matrix* that connected the individual *Universes*). [From this point onward, the "top-level" of *creation* (*&tc.*) is always represented by a *"star"* or *"stars."*]

In addition to the individual *Home Universes*, there were also *"Shared Universes"* that one could go to and experience meetings with others—usually for "games" and various forms of "entertainment." Some of these were like *"Story-Universes"* that functioned as immersive movie theatres. They followed prescribed "scripts" but were laid out as an entire *Universe* (similar to the reality experience everyday on Earth).

When we consider its origins: the *Home Universe Matrix* was *constructed* to prevent *Alpha-Spirits* from interfering with each other's *creations*. But, without any *enforced agreements* on this condition, it was not long before individuals were "hacking" into other *Home Universes* and *creating* problems. We then *agreed* that *Alpha-Spirits* that "broke the rules" needed to be *punished*.

So, we collectively came up with an idea that has forever since been the basis of our ongoing *spiritual degradation*: we designed the first *Implanted Penalty Universes*, or "prisons."

During the *"Home Universe"* era, *Alpha-Spirits* were still quite immune to any use of *"force."* There wasn't really anything you could "do" to someone else. However, large groups began working together to *create* a *complex* series of *"sub-Universes"* that might make someone feel "unpleasant" or "unhappy" while confined there for a while. We all *agreed* this was a good idea to use on the "bad guys"—but no one expected that they, themselves, would ever be forced into experiencing such *"prisons."*

A more complete treatment of *"Implanted Universes"* requires its own *Systemology Level-7 AT Course* manual (particularly where it concerns *defragmenting* with *systematic processing*). For present purposes, we at least shall say that these *Penalty-Prison Universes Implants* installed the primary "emotional curve" (such as you find on the lower half of the *Beta-Awareness Scale*) that we are still the *effect* of today.

These *"Implants"* also used all kinds of interesting *"symbols"* and *"construct-forms"* and *"body types"* to lay in "degrading" *concepts* and *ideals*. Many *low-level* *"goals"* —such as "sex" and "eating" — were *implanted* to limit the *spiritual abilities* of a *"criminal"* —and keep their *attention* suspended on experiencing the activities within the *"Prison-Universe"* (or else they might "break free" of it). These were "*actual*" *Universes*; and the experiences were "real" enough for us to eventually continue these *reality-agreements* as our own *creation*.

At first, these little "*prisons*" didn't seem to have much effect on reducing the amount of *conflict*. But there is a long period of time where we kept throwing *Alpha-Spirits* through the routines so repeatedly that we began to more *compulsively dramatize* the "degradation" of these "*prison*" experiences in our everyday lives.

As mentioned previously, the first "*Shared-Universes*" for "*games*" were also *constructed* during the *Home Universe* era. These started off quite basic, but eventually evolved into more *complex*—rougher and tougher—arenas. The most *complex* of these is referred to simply as the "*Games-Universe*" and it took place on a *game-field* that very closely resembles modern-day *Earth*. [It is no coincidence that our modern *Earth* is a *"prison planet copy"* of the *original Earth*; it is meant to suspend our *attention* in *confusion* and *restimulation*.]

The *original Earth* was intended for the *ultimate "Games-Universe"* (not a *prison*)— and we each spent a lot of time *playing* this *"game."* The primary component of the *game* pertained to *"personality-persona-packages."* By this we mean the *"Artist"* or the *"Scientist,"* &tc. These roles each had specific *characteristics* that affected how they *interrelated* (or *interacted*) with other roles. [Some essential information on this area is given in *PC Lesson-12, "Games & Universes."* See also: *Systemology Level-7 AT Course* manual *"Games, Goals & Purposes."*]

Participation in the *Games* became the most popular activity for *Alpha-Spirits.* They also began to draw more and more *spectators* (onlookers). The real *fragmentation* (at this time) concerned the *implant-*

ing (*conditioning*) required for one to *enter* the *Games-Universe*—because we all went through that "*screen*" innumerable times. It was not a permanent place; we were not confined to it. We could easily just *decide* to leave the *Games* at any point and return to our *Home Universe* to *consider* our *playtime* experience. Later, we could just go back to the *Games* and try something different (passing through the *implant-screen* each time).

For those who "broke the rules" (or cheated), the *Penalty Universes* were there.

But individuals always found a way around the "rules"—so the "*barriers*" or "*restrictions*" were made increasingly more "*solid*" (they were imbued with more *energetic-mass*). Eventually we began to develop a *preference*—associations or attachments—for certain "*roles*" and "*forms.*" And more of the *Home Universe Matrix* (*upper-level Universe*) was starting to resemble (be in *reality-agreement* with) the *Games-Universe*.

As more *Alpha-Spirits* were able to "cheat" or even sidestep *conditioning effects*, more of the *creations* from the *Penalty-Universes* were incorporated into the *Games-Universe*. These were intended to establish additional *barriers* (*restrictions*) to the *Games*. Many of these *constructs* were also requested as "prizes" by various "winners"—where they could then be more permanently "displayed" like "trophies" after the *Games* (back in the *upper-level Universe Matrix*). This then caused the *Home Universe Matrix* to take on more qualities of (or be in *reality-agreement* with) the *Penalty-Universes*, too.

All of these factors contributed to an increased degree of "*reality-agreement*" between the *Penalty-Universes*, the *Games-Universe* and the *Home Universe Matrix*. It is unclear what specifically triggered the events that came next. But, the commonality of *reality-agreement* between too many *creations*—or *"anchor-points"*—bridging between *Universes* could cause them to *"collapse together."* And this is basically what happened.

You might have already had the *"top-level sea of stars"* display *"turned on"* when it happened; or you might have sensed something very strange happening, and turned it *"on"* to investigate. You may have even been in the *Games-Universe* on the *original Earth* at the time. In any case: the *"stars and sky begin to fall."* Each of our *Home Universes* collapses into the (original) *Games-Earth*. The collision builds such an *energetic-mass* that the *original Earth* literally explodes, sending pieces of our own *Universe* scattered through the *"cosmos."*

This *incident* represents our first significant *imprint* for *"loss"* and *"grief."* Everything we have endured since has resulted in accumulation of *fragmentation* built up on *this incident*. The *collapse* or *loss* of *Home Universe* is quite basic to each of us. It is quite difficult to eliminate all the residual *effects* this *incident* has had on us ever since—but it is the direction toward which we travel when applying *systematic processing.*

This *incident* includes a lot of "lightning-energy" filling up *Space*, while our personal *creations* begin to decay and crumble to dust. *Home Universe* was no longer separate from all other existences and became affected by those other *reality-agreements.* With the *"Collapse-of-Universes,"* the *agreed-upon* "laws" and "parameters" of the *Games-Universe* and *Penalty-Universes* became a part of the *Universe* you were in.

THE GAME CONTINUES

The new *"Games-Universe"* became the first real *compulsively agreed-upon "Shared-Universe"* where you (as an individual *Alpha-Spirit*) could no longer maintain *full control* of the *creation* of *reality*. The *Universe* had greatly "expanded" with the residual of all prior *creations*. With the incorporation of *Penalty-Universe constructs* and *agreements*, the *Game* had also become quite "twisted" and "degrading."

Although we were still *god-like Alpha-Spirits* that were immune to *"force,"* the reduction in *creative ability* left us quite *fragmented*. For one thing: we couldn't be "hurt," but our *creations* could. In the *Home Universe* era, we could simply *create* something again; but with the *loss* of *Home Universe*, it became obvious that we could now *"lose"* something. This affected our *consideration* of *"having"* or "*havingness.*" Suddenly, "*having for us*" meant "*not having for others.*"

Individual *Alpha-Spirits* chose remote areas of the *Universe* and "staked their claim" on the *Space* by placing some kind of *creations* there—even if it were only a "nebulous cloud" or a "suspended picture." We were still able to "*create,*" but it was all now within the confines of the formerly established *reality-agreements.*

When mutual "*game activity*" resumed again, it began quite tame—more "intellectual"—with everyone still getting over the initial shock and trauma of the *collapse.* But we are quite "resilient" beings; and it did not take long before more and more of the *Universe* became "business as usual." By this, we mean that the structure of events that we have described so far in this manual is the basic *blueprint* or *systematic pattern* behind the events that have continued to take place on the *Backtrack* ever since.

Here, once again, we find ourselves having to *confront* those "undesirable" individuals that seem to do nothing but *create* trouble. Basically, we want them "out" of the *Game* altogether. Naturally, we all *decided* to get together and *construct* a new lower-level *Universe* that could hold the "criminals" in such a way that they wouldn't just get out and make more trouble again. Some new "mechanism" was required.

The residual *Penalty Universe* materials (*reality-agreements* and *Implants*) were collected and strung together, rather like a "carousel" surrounding a "treadmill." Up until this point, the *Alpha-Spirit* did not experience any real sensation of "*motion.*" This new "mechanism" impressed the original *Penalty-Universe* "*goals*" in an endlessly streaming line of dwindling or descending conditions.

A positive "*goal*" was paired with its opposite (negative characteristic), which would then lead to the next positive, on and on perpetually. The *Implant* basically encouraged those entering this new *"lower-Universe"* to focus on *"doing each other in,"* rather than placing any *attention* on trying to "escape" (or leaving).

This is the first time that a *Prison-Universe* was actually intended to be a *permanent* solution for handling undesirable individuals. There is no way to "kill" an *immortal spirit*; so all you can do is "exile" one.

At first, the *Implanting* used to get an *Alpha-Spirit* into the *"prison"* and keep them there is not very effective. Part of keeping the individual there requires having "interesting" and "distracting" things to occupy them. But, as the individual keeps escaping and then getting pushed back in through the *Implanting*, the repeated exposure begins to have a real effect. As more time passes, more individuals end up in the *"Prison Universe"* at a particular time, so the *game-conditions* there become even more interesting and interactive.

As with our previous *"lower-level prison constructs,"* no one ever expects themselves to get thrown in; but it ultimately happens to nearly everyone. Sometimes even as a joke or prank, or simply because it's there. After enough times, the *Alpha-Spirit* develops an interest (and then an attachment) to the *lower-order* "motions" and "sensations" that are attached to the *lower-level Universe.* An individual can even develop a tendency to *want* to go there for the "sensation" (much like a "drug")—and then gets to realizing they don't like it anymore, remembers they're in a *"prison,"* and starts focusing on "getting out" again.

There are always those who remain in the *"upper-level"* Universe (out of "prison") in *control* (as the *winning leaders*). Still, there comes a time when so much of the population has been relocated to a *"lower-*

order" Universe, that the *"upper-level" Universe* no longer remains interesting (or inhabited) enough to be sustainable. In many ways the *upper-Universe* begins to "contract" and "decay."

The last group still remaining there eventually decides that they have no choice but to descend into the *lower-Universe.* [This general pattern of activity continues through the remaining sequence of *condensing Universes.*]

Additionally, the last group that has remained out of the *"prison-system"* is able to descend "in style." They have not been subjected to the same *conditioning-Implants* as the other "prisoners" have. In each cycle of *condensing-Universes,* these "leaders" are able to retain the "technology" and "knowledge" of the previous *Universe* and descend upon (and "invade") the *lower-level* population as *"gods."* [In this case, we can see many parallels with the *"Anunnaki"* of *Mesopot-*

amian history, as explored in *"Mardukite Zuism"* materials.]

The primary tactic these *"invader-gods"* often use requires *constructing* a *"False Jewel of Knowledge."* The experience of this subsequent *"Implanting"* is actually *"earned"* and/or *"fought for."* It provides the illusion of what we might consider *"religious/spiritual enlightenment,"* but it really *conditions* an individual to be a more willing slave of the *"gods."* In extreme cases, it produces bizarre *"religious ideals"* and *"fanatics."*

In this first instance after the *Games-Universe*, the *"gods"* descended upon the *prison-population* and incited a *"Holy War."* While there had always been *"conflict"* among individuals, this marked the first occurrence of *"organized warfare."* And it was orchestrated by *"higher beings"* simply to *control* a *"lower population"* under the guise of *"religion."* While these *"gods"* did exercise a tremendous power and authority, they were never able to fully control the population. There was a revolt; they were overthrown; kingdoms were laid to waste.

After the endless waves of *"Holy War,"* the *creations* and *conditions* of the *Universe* was left in ruin. Half the population was *"insane"* from *religious-implanting* and the remainder were *turbulently-charged* from the *counter-measures* and *misemotion* connected to fighting against the others. They *decided* that these "evil characters" (the *"gods"* and their *"fanatics"*) that unleashed the *creation* of *"War"* were unforgivable and had to be gotten rid of. And so we continued the patterned cycle of *creating lower-level "Prison Universes"* — and we took turns being the "good guys" and the "bad guys" and throwing each other *down lower and lower.*

"THE SYMBOLS UNIVERSE"

To be *systematic*, we refer to this newly constructed *prison* as the *"Symbols Universe"* (though none of these existences were really given proper names). The *"transfer-point"* or *"entry-point"* *Implant* required an *Alpha-Spirit* to "compartmentalize" *hidden pieces* of themselves—the *"spiritual machinery"* we *compulsively create*, yet *"hide"* from ourselves. [*PC Lesson-14.*] This is the initial origin of the *"Mind-System"* as we know it—and what is poorly termed the *"subconscious."*

Here we find *"hidden parts"* of ourselves able to be *imprinted* upon, which can then generate "sensations" and "considerations" *reactively* (*automatically*) when in the presence of some *"symbolic"* stimulation. By this, we mean a sort of *"Reactive Control Center"* that triggers a *stimulus-response reaction* to a *"symbol"* or *"mental image picture"* that merely represents something actual. For the first time: *symbols* have *significance*. You couldn't affect the being; but now you could get a being to affect themselves by showing them something (particularly those *"symbols"* from the *Penalty-Universes*).

The *"games"* and *Implants* from this era primarily concerned *imprinted symbols*. Fighting opponents would direct streams of reoccurring *symbols* at one another. This didn't really do much at first, but as individuals wanted their *symbols* to produce greater effects, they went into greater *agreement* with the *imprinting*, and the *symbols* took on greater *"solidity."*

The big concern an *Alpha-Spirit* had at this time was how to prevent unwanted *symbols* from being pushed directly into one's *viewpoint* (*Awareness*) and automatically triggering some undesirable *effect*. Our solution to this was to *create* "substitutions" in place of our *actual presence*, to act as *communication-relays* for whatever we might *perceive*. As a result, you find *Alpha-Spirits* start *deciding* to "dampen" or "lessen" their own *telepathic abilities*. [And it is important to note here: in spite of any conditions that may have encouraged it, the *actual* "lessening" of one's own *ability* is something that only the individual, themselves, could make happen.]

When the final *"upper-level"* group descended, they had *constructed* a new *"Pyramid Trap" Implant*. As usual, it utilized *"higher"* knowledge and technology carried forth from earlier *Universes*. This *construct* resembled a gigantic *Pyramid* with an open door; hollow inside, except for something fascinating at its center that most likely resembled *The Jewel* (but in appearance only). As soon as the *Alpha-Spirit* is drawn inside, the door closes behind.

Within the *Pyramid* are *128* layers of

"walls" or "facets" —one for each of the 64 original *Penalty-Universes* (plus an inverted version of the same). Each *wall* is saturated with *symbols* from that particular *Penalty-Universe*. The *Alpha-Spirit* begins to work through this sequence, working from the center outward. But each time there is a layer they can't *confront*, they end up back at the center again.

The *Pyramid Trap* impresses an illusion that much more "time" is passing during these endless attempts than actually is. This starts to embed *fragmentation* about *Time*—and this develops into sensations of being anxious about "getting things done" or "missing out on other things." The *Alpha-Spirit* starts to experience a sense of "desperation" that previously had never existed.

Once the *Alpha-Spirit* is "sufficiently" desperate, the "*invader-gods*" pull the individual out of the *Implant-Construct* and keep its *Awareness* in a state of suspension, while they are blasted from each side with streams of *Penalty-Universe Symbols*. The effect of this is much stronger than when first entering the *Symbols Universe*. After the *Pyramid Trap*, these waves of repeated *symbols* override the additional "communication-relays" the individual set up. The *symbols* now operated as "*terminals*" for the individual's *spiritual machinery*.

Of course, there was a revolution (as there always is). The "*invader-gods*" were overrun by the masses and thrown into their own *Traps*. And more elaborate *Traps* were *constructed*. Unlike prior *systems*, the *Symbols Universe* had developed into a quite *complex civilization*. This is the point in our history when *Alpha-Spirits* became *fragmented* enough to require (and demand) *creation* of a "*formal government*" and "*a council*."

Here too, we see the first "*large cities*" and "*police forces*." In this era, we also find the original archetype for a centralized city, known as *"Alpha Prime."*

The level of *"solidity"* experienced in the *Symbols Universe* is still nothing like what we have today. Existence mainly consisted of *"thought planes"* — two-dimensional pictures suspended in *Space* that are experienced three-dimensionally when you "step into" them. Doing so would require, at least temporarily, *creating* a *form* for your *Awareness* (*sense of Beingness*) to "be there" and interact with whatever/whoever it was.

Alpha-Spirits were still "disembodied" as a *Beingness*; but they could sense the presence of one another and would even flash certain *symbols* — "signs" or "sigils" or "signatures" — to *identify* themselves. Communication had become *"symbolic"* rather than *"telepathic."* We did not yet inhabit the kind of *fleshy bodies* we do today, but we began to *identify* with *symbolic-creations* more often. And if we had to appear before the *Council* (or in "court"), the *police force* would *enforce* you to "appear" in an expected *form*.

The Council existed for most of the *Symbols Universe* era. Members served in rotation. Each of us has likely maintained some position on one of these *Councils*. Specific "regimes" were constantly being overthrown and replaced. This, too, was part of the *games* of the *Universe* — "betrayal" and "treachery" against other *council-members*. This was also the first great *"machine-building"* age. Whenever someone would visit one of the *thought-planes*, their own *creations* (*postulates*) tended to alter it; so *"machines"* would reset it afterward.

When the final group of "invader-gods" descended to the *Symbols Universe*, they were met by an advanced and sophisticated *civilization*. The *Council* had already begun using *Prison-Universes* on their own criminals, but then the convict would spend forever working out the details of the *Implants*, escape, and then work to imprison the ones that had imprisoned them. Therein, the cycle had already repeated; but with each time, the *Implants* became more complex. Learning new ways to "escape" again, simply became part of the *game.*

"*Sensation Pools*" were another new development during this era. "Signals" from one's experience in a *thought-plane* would prompt their *invisible machinery* to draw "*sensation*" from these "*pools.*" This provided the *sense* of *emotion* and even *pain*; but the actual *sensation* was drawn from a "hidden source" and not the (apparent) *symbol* that prompted it. This is when we began to "*misidentify*" the "*sources*" of things. And this is where our story begins to take a turn.

The *Symbols Universe* would have been the last step taken when we still retained the *Awareness* and *spiritual ability* enough to collectively "stop" our further descent. The last members of the *Symbols Universe* got very interested in the activities of one of their little *"prison"* sequences again—and they never returned. There is likely no longer anyone there to "pull" us all out of here. None of the other *"prison sequences"* went more than *two* levels below the *Symbols Universe*. The present *Physical Universe* is now *four sub-levels* deep—and the next one below us is *already* in *operation*. We're likely really in it for keeps now; for all the marbles.

"THOUGHT" & "ENERGY"

Directly beneath the *Symbols Universe*, everyone ends up in the most *complex prison* made during the previous era. We refer to this as the *"Thought Universe"* because its inhabitants considered themselves as *"Thought Beings"*—but really, they were *"Energy Beings,"* as opposed to the *"Body Beings"* (of the next *lower-level* prison).

The *transfer-point* or *entry-incident* leading down into the *"Thought Universe"* consists of a four-dimensional *"spiral staircase"* that appears to extend infinitely. The *construct Implants* a "postulate" that: an *Alpha-Spirit* (as a *Beingness*) is an *"energy-unit"*—and therefore, can be "hit" by *energy* and *force*. As one descends the *"spiral staircase,"* the sense of *imprinting* (using cues from *The Jewel of Knowledge*) becomes more "vivid" as it "accumulates" progressively as *fragmentation*.

During the *Thought Universe* era, an *Alpha-Spirit* identifies its *Beingness* with a specific fixed *"energetic-body"* for the first time. Of course, it was really like an *"energy-sphere"* (rather than a more material form)—but the individual is now *"located"* in *Space* (as a specific *anchor-point* moving about the *universal matrix*). As

83

soon as we naively *agreed* to the *reality* of *energy-bodies,* we could be trapped and hurt by *energy,* and "pushed around" and conditioned by *force.* This *"thought-energy"* state of *Beingness* was still far above what those below in more *"material bodies"* experienced; but we had far descended from our native *god-like* state.

Because quite *fragmented* individuals inhabited the *Thought Universe,* a *sub-level prison* was *constructed* rather quickly. It became the first *"physical"* Universe, though much less condensed than *this* present *Physical Universe.* In order to avoid confusion, we will refer to that one as the *"Conflicts Universe,"* because that is the *only* thing which took place at that level of existence. We could refer to this *conflict* as the *"Thought-Energy"* (or *"Mind-Matter"*) *Wars;* fought between *"Thought-Energy Beings"* and the *lower-level "Material-Body Beings."*

At the time, the *Conflict Universe* developed two-levels below the *Symbols Uni-verse* (which was still inhabited by its "elite"). Other *Symbols Universe* "prisons" that had subdivided before, but eventually this *Thought-Universe to Conflicts-Universe* sequence is where everyone ended up.

This *War* went on for a very long time. We switched sides often: the *Body Beings* escaping and becoming *Thought Beings;* *Thought Beings* being caught or imprisoned and existing as a *Body Being* — and each type fighting against the other. Even the *beings* from the *Symbols Universe* started getting involved in the *War* (showing up as "*gods*" as usual).

As the *Symbols Universe* emptied out, both the *Thought Universe* and *Conflicts Universe* began to expand. Toward the end of the *War*, all of the increased "*crossings*" back and forth between *Universes* required more *transfer-points* (and *anchor-points*) in common — until the two *Univer-*

ses finally *collapsed* together. The result was a "layered" *Universe*, with a "*material plane*" (of "*material bodies*") and a "*thought plane*" (where you went in between "*material lives*"). We were still quite aware of the distinction between these two states; that our "*energetic bodies*" continued to "reincarnate" in *material forms*.

After the *Wars* and the *collapse*, the "*material plane*" appeared very much like various "continents" or "landscapes" simply floating through *Space*. There is a long period of redevelopment and building new *civilizations*, but given the former events, everyone was quite hesitant to *construct* another *Prison-Universe*. But *conflict* was inevitable; as individuals just couldn't seem to leave each other well enough alone.

We begin to see more *Implanting* efforts taking place from *within* the *Universe* (rather than a "*prison*"), in order to make others "slaves" or "good citizens"—but in any case, to generally fall in line. *False data* from *The Jewel of Knowledge* continued to be *dramatized* as we used heavier and heavier *conditioning* on each other. Because of the identification of our *Beingness* at this point: it was possible to capture an *"energy-body"* and *force* it into a *"material-body,"* only to "kill it off" with a certain condition, and then do it again repeatedly.

Toward the end of this era, a certain "group" formed with the *intention* of bringing a unified *"peace"* to the *Universe*, once and for all. They established a centralized government and a centralized city (similar to *"Alpha Prime"*) that could maintain *control* over the entire population by establishing a standard *social structure* or *society*, to which everybody would be subject to. And so, the *"Magic Kingdom"* was born.

THE MAGIC KINGDOM & UNIVERSE

The *"Magic Kingdom"* emerged from the remnants of the *Thought-Conflicts Universe* collapse, near the end of that era. It was built on one of the "floating continents"—a grandiose "castle" beside a lake and surrounded by forest. [The archetypal imagery is strangely similar to the iconic scenery often used in "logos" and "title cards" by the Walt Disney Company—which they also refer to as the "Magic Kingdom."] It is the first real visual *imprint* of a *"floating castle," "cloud-castle,"* and/or *"castle in the sky."*

Creators of the *Magic Kingdom* had salvaged four-dimensional technology from previous *Universes.* This allowed the inside of the *"castle-construct"* to essentially extend indefinitely with three-dimensional hallways and corridors that curved slightly at four-dimensional angles. This means it had the potential *Space* for everyone in the *Universe* to live there. [A reader might immediately call to mind some of the statements made by *Jesus Christ* concerning a *"heavenly kingdom"* and *"mansion with many rooms."*]

The *Magic Kingdom* was a *"pyramid-society"* based on "classes." New citizens entered the *system* as "servants," and then others would "move up" in their "status." In many ways, one's "privileges" and "class" really depended on how *early* they joined up. And when it seemed like the *Magic Kingdom* was going to "take over" the *Universe*, there was a surge of new willing recruits entering in with the expectation that they would eventually become *"overseers"* as the population continued to grow.

As with any *pyramid-based* social (or organizational) *system* developed ever since, there is at least some sense of "slavery" inherent in any position except the *top-level*—and of course, as the majority of the *Universe* entered into the *Magic Kingdom* and filled positions, it seemed that the hope for *later* recruits to elevate one's status disappeared. New individuals stopped coming. And here we find "legions" of "*winged-warriors*" and "*mystic-knights on flying-horses*" on missions to expand the *Magic Kingdom* by forcibly enslaving the remaining population in the *Universe*.

Once every *Alpha-Spirit* and every *creation* in the *Universe* had been collected and incorporated into the *Magic Kingdom*, the *system collapsed*. The "*castle-infrastructure*" was still there but things were no longer functioning; operations had become too *militant* and *totalitarian* to sustain the *civilization* as it stood. Revolts by the *lower-class* masses—who held the advantage only by their sheer numbers—overthrew *higher-classes*.

Everyone *realized* that this "*mode of operat-*

ing" would ultimately lead to a *systematic* catastrophe on a *cosmic scale* if these cycles of *enslavement* continued in this way. There needed to be a "place" to put an *upper-class* when they were over-thrown. Yet, by this point, we had collectively understood some of the mistakes that were continuously taking place on our *"descent"* — and a typical *"prison-construct"* would likely mean risking something like the previous *"Thought-Conflict" Wars.* We could at least all *agree* that no one wanted to see that happen.

When the next *"prison"* was *created*, the place needed to be pleasant enough to want to stay there.

If the "prisoners" could actually be happy, they wouldn't be interested in trying to escape back to the *Magic Kingdom.* In fact, if it were reminiscent of both the *Magic Kingdom* and *original Earth* of the *Games-Universe*, combined with an *Implanted-Goal "To Enjoy,"* this new *"prison"* might actually be a nice place to live. So, that is exactly what was *constructed*—and the *"Magic Universe"* was brought into *existence*.

Materials for previous *Systemology Levels* did not distinguish between the *Magic Kingdom* (of the *Conflicts-Universe*) and the *Magic Universe*. There are many similarities between the two. But, the *Magic Universe* is the *"Astral Otherworld"* or *"Fairyland" Universe* that immediately precedes our *present Physical Universe*. However, it is *not* the *"thought plane"* we return to in between our physical lifetime incarnations.

An *Implant-construct* resembling a *"volcano"* served as the *transfer-point* from the *Magic Kingdom* to the *Magic Universe*. An individual would ascend a pathway to the top; the whole time, passing by *"statues"* representing the *Penalty-Prison Universe "symbols"* or *"terminals"* (as was common to these *transfer-points*). When they got to the *"peak"* or *"mouth"* of the *volcano*, they were thrown in.

It didn't take very long before waves of individuals were willingly jumping into the *volcano* just to get "reborn" in the *Magic Universe*. The *Entry-Incident* at the start of our experience in the *Magic Universe* includes a *"Wizard"* riding a *"magic carpet"* over toward you from an *"Arabian-styled ship"* (or *"dhow"*). He is carrying a *"glowing ball"* (or *"orb"*) between his slightly uplifted hands.

Bodies in the *Magic Universe* are, in appearance, very much like the *"physical bodies"* we are familiar with in *this Physical Universe*. One key difference is that in the *Magic Universe*, the "internal structure" of a *Body* is entirely composed of *"energy centers"* (or *"chakras"*) as opposed to *"solid genetic organs."* Today, we would refer to this *"body"* used in the *Magic Universe* as the *"Astral Body."* In fact, many of the concepts in modern and ancient *myst-*

icism really originate, and are far more relevant, in the *Magic Universe.*

For example: the inspiration behind the design of the *Magic Universe* included the events that *collapsed* the former *Universes* and *structured* a *two-layered* "Thoughts plus Conflicts" *Universe.* Therefore, in the *Magic Universe*, we find a *"material/physical layer"* plus a *"heavenly layer"* (above) and a *"demonic layer"* (below).

Among these three "*layers,*" virtually every "fantasy," "fairy tale," "religious," and "mythological" manifestation conceivable, *existed.* Even *disembodied beings* would *visibly* move around for a while, using their former "*Energy-Body*" manifestation from the *Conflicts-Universe*, before reincarnating as another "*Astral Body.*"

The *Implanted Game-Goal* governing the *Magic Universe* was "To Enjoy." At the time, the lowest *energy-center* (or "*chakra*") of the *Astral Body* was in the *"genital-region."* Much of the hedonistic activity here involved *"sex."* Anything resembling *"foods"* or *"consumable substances"* was *created* purely for *sensation* or *effect*. [An even lower *energy-center* around the *"rectum"* was added to the *Astral Body* before entering the present *Physical Universe*; but in the *Magic Universe*, there was no need to eliminate *"body waste."*]

The *Game* of the *Magic Universe* included *upper-level roles* of *"gods"* and *"goddesses," "angels"* and *"demons,"* in the *layers* surrounding the *material plane*. Although the main purpose was *"To Enjoy,"* we still find individuals trying to get the upper-hand over others, or *condition* one another to be *"good"* (according to their own definitions).

We eventually find the remaining population coming down *willingly* from the *Magic Kingdom*, armed with the technology and knowledge of former *Universes* in order to secure those upper-most *roles* and *positions* in the *Magic Universe*. [Some imagery from these events even includes *"great castles" descending* from the *skies*.] The *games* and *conflicts* of the *Magic Universe* went on for a long time before everyone *agreed* to *construct* a *lower-level prison* again. And so, this *present Physical Universe* we are currently in, was built.

THE PHYSICAL UNIVERSE

The *transfer-point* and *entry-incident* regarding the shift between the *Magic Universe* and *this Physical Universe* is first introduced to a *Seeker* in *PC Lesson-12*, *"Games & Universes,"* as we shall excerpt from here.

This *Physical Universe* was *created* as a place to penalize, exile, or otherwise imprison, the criminals and maladjusted individuals from the *Magic Universe*. At first, we would all "escape" back to the *Magic Universe*—so there have been many repeated *entry-incidents* (*Implanting*) into *this Physical-Universe*.

After a legal sentencing, an individual finds themselves being "drawn down" to *descend* a *"spiral of pillars"* into a Grecian/Roman-style *"pool."* The archetypal *Penalty-Prison Universe* symbols/ *terminals* are each on one of the *pillars*. Whatever *Beings* are present (above/ around the *pool*) use their *energy* to "push down" upon the individual as well— thereby also participating in the *"implanting-incident"* that ensues.

This *implanting-incident* does not contain much *"pain"* (or *"force"*). It takes place in a *"mini-verse"* designed (in the *Magic Universe*) to be *"aesthetically-beautiful,"* so as to hold one's *attention* and eventually draw the individual into the *Physical Universe*. Any real *"turbulence"* incited by the *incident* itself, is merely a sense of *"loss"* (over leaving the *Magic Universe*) or mise-motion regarding *"exile"*—or of feeling *"pushed out."*

There are really two parts to this *incident*. In the *first* part: an individual finds themselves essentially floating in a *"void-like space"* with a sensation similar to being *"under water."* They eventually see a *"golden light"* in the distance—it glimmers and radiates like a sunburst. [The *"False Jewel"* of this *incident*.]

Once the individual's *attention* is fixed upon it, they are "drawn" toward it with increasing speed. This *"golden light"* is a *symbol/terminal* (*"Object-Item"*) attached to the first *"Implanted Goal"* of an entire sequence (consisting of *36* "Goals" or *"archetypes"*). [In this case, the first one is: *"To Be Godlike."*]

Each *"Goal"* is introduced and *identified* with a particular *"Object-Item"* (in order to *communicate* and *embed/encode* its significance). The *"Goals" are* named, but the titles are *sensed* (or *intuited*) rather than expressed in words. [We only *approximate* their meaning with *Human* language for *study* and *processing*.]

As the individual is "drawn in and through" each *"Object-Item,"* the *"Goal"* is *identified* and understood. This continues with increasing speed through the remaining sequence—informing *what* the *"Goals" are.* It sets up the *second* part of the *incident*, when this *"Goals-Sequence"* is *implanted* again with more *significance.*

In the *second* part: the individual emerges from the final *"Object-Item"* in the sequence (a *"pyramid"* associated with the Goal: *"To Be Enduring"*) and finds themselves facing an *"amphitheater stage"* in the distance ahead of them. [This *incident* is sometimes referred to as the *"Heaven Implant,"* because the scenery (of this *second* part) includes a stereotypical *heavenly "trumpet-blasting-angels-in-the-clouds"* atmosphere that *Humans* are *implanted* to "expect" for their *after-life* (or more correctly: *"between-lives"* period).] There is often the sense of being surrounded by many others and everyone rushing up toward the *"stage."*

A *trumpet-horn* blasts, and a sharp *snapping-crackle* (like the *pierce of thunder*), to get your *attention* right before any "command-line" is given. The first *command-line* is from an unseen *source* (to get the *"pageant"* started)—*"Only One Will Survive."* Again, the *horn* blasts, the *snap-crackles* happen, and the second *command-line* emerges—*"To Be The One Who Survives, You Must Be Superior To All Others."* This seems to settle the crowd down and all *attention* becomes focused on the stage where a *"pageant-skit"* ensues.

The *blasts* and *snaps* are heard as a new "character" (each representing one of the *"Goals"*) comes on the *stage* to speak *three* *"command-lines."* Only one "character" is on *stage* at a time. They always enter from one side of the *stage* (your right) and exit the other (your left). There is a *procession* or *sequence* taking place, so the "characters" tend to *look* in a particular direction when referring to the *next* (or the *previous*) "character."

When the *final* "character" (*An Enduring Being*) completes their reference to the *first* (*A Godlike Being*), the *implanting-incident* ends with "waves of blackness" before the individual finds themselves with fixed *viewpoints* in *this Physical Universe* (*Beta-Existence*). Unlike previous *Universes*, the *Space* here is "dark." And while there are many *entry-points* in this *local Universe*, the most current one is the *Horsehead Nebula* (*Orion*).

[The *110* "*command-items*" of this *Implant-Platform* are given in *PC Lesson-12*; and the basic significance for each is "*processed out*" as described in *PC Lesson-11*. Descriptive material (as found in this present *AT Course Manual*) simply helps in "*Spotting*" and "*connecting with*" (*contacting*) specific *Items* and *Implants* for *processing incidents* on the *Backtrack*. Additional details are to be found in other *AT Course Manuals.*]

The *Implant* strongly reinforces that the individual is entering a *Universe* based on "*force*" and "*effort*." Rather than be able to more freely "*create*" *Energy* and *Matter*, the "*Physical Being*" will now have to apply "*force against force*" and "*effort against effort*," using a "*Physical Body*" to *create* and *build*, using only the existing "materials" already provided for them in *this Universe*.

The fundamental *Game-Goal* of *this Physical Universe* is "*To Survive*." In the absence of *true knowledge* about *who* or *what* we really are, all of our *attention*, *energy* and *efforts* become preoccupied with *material survival*. It is the ultimate *spiritual distraction* and *spirit-trap*: to trick/convin-

102

ce an *immortal being* of the *"need to survive."* The individual is continuously *conditioned* to both require the assistance of *others*, yet simultaneously be in competition with them—which safeguards against the masses coming together and "breaking" the *Game*.

Activity and *creation* in *this Physical Universe* pertains almost exclusively to *"material technologies."* When the final *upperlevel "Kings"* and *"Wizards"* of the *Magic Universe* decided that the *"real game"* was now *down here*, they were certain to retain *upper-level* knowledge of *all* "advanced technologies" relevant to *this* Universe. They descended and began constructing *planet-sized "cities"* and gigantic *"spaceships."*

It did not take long before large *organized societies* began making slaves of the population—and eventually such things as a *"Galactic Empire"* developed. As a result of large-scale *"power struggles"* to maintain such an *"Empire,"* the center of *this Galaxy* was *collapsed* into a *"black-hole,"* serving as the *transfer-point* to the next *lower Prison-Universe* (already built). [From the little we know of this next level down, it is nowhere a *Seeker* wants to end up if they still hope for *Ascension.*]

Entire waves of *"invader-gods"* entered into the *Physical Universe.* It would only take a small group of *"Kings"* and *"Wizards"* to capture an entire planetary population, take them back up to the *Magic Universe* for *"advanced training"* (and additional *Implanting*) before collectively returning here again as a *"better-abled"* massive *"legion"* or *"fleet."*

The *Magic Universe* still exists; it has not *collapsed.* It is rather abandoned, however, and is likely *contracting* and *deteriorating* even as you read these words. There are a few of us who have been, until relatively recently, still *transitioning* between *Universes* more fluidly. We have known of a few *"Ascended Masters"* in our recorded *Earth-history*, but the last mass wave of *"invader-gods"* left the *Magic Universe* (and descended to *this* one) approximately *10,000 years ago*. Not too surprisingly, a few of them even show up in the *most ancient writings* that we still have access to on this planet.

OUR CURRENT SITUATION

Of course, things are more *complex* than what is described in this narrative. The fact *this Physical Universe* seems so *"solid"* and so immune to our *"thoughts"* (as an influential *force*), suggests that its whole *existence* is set up, *perceived*, and interacted with, entirely "indirectly." Keep in mind that we have carried all of the *fragmentation* and *spiritual machinery* with us (from experiences in previous *Universes*) into *present-time*. While it has been kept primarily *hidden*, it is the *"spiritual baggage"* that *resurfaces* in *systematic processing* so that we can *confront* it and be rid of it. We must unburden ourselves of its "weight" in order to *Ascend*.

Although *"organic life"* comes in many forms, the *"genetic-vehicles"* or *"Bodies"* preferred by *Alpha-Spirits* in *this Physical Universe* are *"humanoid"* in appearance—though not necessarily *"Human."* By this we mean *two arms, two legs, &tc.* This pattern is something we have carried with us here; developed as part of the *basic structure* that we have now come to progressively—and *compulsively—identify* with *as* our *Beingness*.

The *entire pattern* of our *descent* is embedded in this total *consideration* of *Beingness*; a *structure* of cumulatively *hidden communication-relays*, requiring our *Awareness* to essentially pass through *seven-plus-one* *"veils," "gates,"* or *"thresholds,"* of entire *Universes*, in order to *perceive* something as *solid*—and as *condensed*—as the *reality* of *this Physical Universe.* When we plot this descent in reverse:

• The *"Genetic Vehicle"* (the *Physical Body* of *this "Physical Universe"*); is maintained by an

• *"Astral Body"* (the now-invisible *etheric* form used in the *"Magic Universe"*); which is generated by a

• *"Spirit Body"* (from the *"Conflicts Universe"*); which is projected by an

• *"Energy Body"* (from the *"Thought Universe"*); which is projected by a

• *"Symbol Body"* (from the *"Symbols Universe"*); which is projected by a

• *"Persona-Mask"* (from the *"Motions/ensations Universe"*); which is projected by a

• *"Basic Object"* (our *playing-piece* from the *"Games Universe"*); which is created by the

• *"Alpha-Spirit"* (still operating) from the *viewpoint* of one's *own "Home Universe."*

The *chronicle* of our *descent* is really our *Map-Key* to *The Way Out*. Of course, the *Map* by itself does not make the *Journey*; nor does a possession of this manuscript alone ensure one's *safe travel*. There are some that have escaped the gravity of *this Universe* and returned to a more *god-like* state. But they tend to fall right back into the same *traps* and *conflicts* again. To all this, we propose that *Systemology* is our best solution to the *endless cycles* and *dwindling spirals* of our continuing *spiritual existence*.

The next lower *prison existence* is already constructed. It is *not this Physical Universe* —but based on the types of inhabitants that typically occupy *this planet*, it is likely that a few "*Humans*" have already been there and back and least once. *This planet* is an actual copy of the *original Earth* (from the *Games Universe*) and it is currently used as a "*prison-planet*" by the present *Galactic* "authorities," keeping us far enough away from the center of the *Galaxy*, where most of the "local" activity actually is. These *physical* "Earth-bodies" are not intended to stray far from *this planet*.

If we were to give it a name, the next *Prison-Universe* might be called the "*Endurance Universe*" or "*Dross Universe*." Its *Space* is incredibly *solid/condensed* in all directions, like a thick *syrup* or *quicksand*. It's primary *Implanted Games-Goal* is: "*To Persist*" or "*To Endure*." At least in the *Physical Universe*, (the *Goal*) "*To Survive*" denotes some flexibility of *action*; but in the next level down, we might just find ourselves—an *Eternal Spiritual Being*—entrapped in that *persisting existence* as a "*rock*" or "*grain of sand*" for a "*Body*." Sounds very unpleasant.

Although this narrative might seem depressing, or portray a hopeless situation, it is really the story of a *god* that forgets who and what they are, but always has the chance it turn in all around again. This story of ours hasn't ended. We are still writing it—still playing at the *games* of *creation*. But we have clearly come to a crossroads; and our *decision* is whether to allow ourselves to continue in the direction we have been headed, or whether to *change* course, and return back up the *Pathway*; retracing our *steps*, working our way *systematically* out of the *traps*—and sharing our treasure-trove of *new creations* with the *"older beings"*—having finally earned our "right" to join them for the first time. This is what we originally had set out to do in the very beginning.

While there are certainly more details available to a *Seeker*: the *Truth of All Things* is no simpler than we have described. This *"Secret Doctrine"* unravels thousands of years of obscure *spiritual traditions*, *mysticism* and *religious belief*. It recovers the real knowledge that other modern efforts to interpret the *Kabbalah* and the *Star-Gates* have failed to unveil. It collects and unifies the underlying truth behind all *Life, Universes* and *Everything*. From *psychology* to *physics*; from *economics* to *politics*; it explains all too bluntly just why conditions are the way they are —and it suggests, quite strongly, the precise *Pathway* that we must follow to find *The Way Out*.

Your next Advanced Training manual is:
"*Games, Goals & Purposes*"

BASIC SYSTEMOLOGY GLOSSARY

actualization : to make actual, not just potential; to bring into full solid Reality; to realize fully in *Awareness* as a "thing."

agreement (reality) : unanimity of opinion of what is "thought" to be known; an accepted arrangement of how things are; things we consider as "real" or as an "is" of "reality"; a consensus of what is real as made by standard-issue (common) participants; what an individual contributes to or accepts as "real"; in *Systemology*, a synonym for "*reality.*"

alpha : the first, primary, basic, superior or beginning of some form; in *Systemology*, referring to the state of existence operating on spiritual archetypes and postulates, will and intention "exterior" to the low-level condensation and solidarity of energy and matter as the 'physical universe' (*beta*).

alpha-spirit : a "spiritual" *Life*-form; the "true" *Self* or I-AM; the *individual*; the spiritual (*alpha*) *Self* that is animating the (*beta*) physical body or "*genetic vehicle*" using a continuous *Lifeline* of spiritual ("*ZU*") energy; an individual spiritual (*alpha*) entity possessing no physical mass or measurable waveform (motion) in the Physical Universe as itself, so it animates the (*beta*) physical body or "*genetic vehicle*" as a catalyst to experience *Self*-determined causality in effect within the *Physical Universe*; a singular unit or point of *Spiritual Awareness* that is *Aware* that it is *Aware*.

alpha thought : the highest spiritual *Self-determination* over creation and existence exercised by an Alpha-Spirit; the Alpha range of pure *Creative Ability* based on direct postulates and considerations of *Beingness*; spiritual qualities comparable to "thought" but originating in Alpha-existence, independently superior to a Mind-System.

ascension : actualized *Awareness* elevated to the point of true "spiritual existence" exterior to *beta existence*. An "Ascended Master" is one who has returned to an incarnation on Earth as an inherently *Enlightened One*, demonstrable in their words and actions; they have the ability to *Self-direct* the "Mind" and "Body" as *Self* (as a "Spirit"); and to maintain consciousness as a personal identity continuum with the same *Self-directed* control and communication of Will-Intention that is exercised, actualized and developed deliberately during one's present incarnation.

associative knowledge : significance or meaning of a facet or aspect assigned to (or considered to have) a direct relationship with another facet; to connect or relate ideas or facets of existence with one another; in traditional systems logic, an equivalency of significance or meaning between facets or sets that are grouped together, such as in *(a + b) + c = a + (b + c)*; in Systemology, erroneous associative knowledge is assignment of the same value to all facets or parts considered as related (even when they are not actually so), such as in *a = a, b = a, c = a* and so forth without distinction.

attention : active use of *Awareness* toward a specific aspect or thing; the act of "attending" with the presence of *Self*; a direction of focus or concentration of *Awareness* along a particular channel or conduit or toward a particular terminal node or communication termination point; the Self-directed concentration of personal energy as a combination of observation, thought-waves and consideration; focused application of *Self-Directed Awareness*.

awareness : the highest sense of-and-as *Self* in knowing and being as I-AM (the *Alpha-Spirit*); the extent of beingness directed as a viewpoint (POV) experienced by *Self* as *Knowingness*.

beta (awareness) : all consciousness activity ("*Awareness*") in the "Physical Universe" (KI,

114

in *Zuism*) or else in *beta-existence*; *Awareness* within the range of the *genetic-body*, including material thoughts, emotional responses and physical motors; personal *Awareness* of physical energy and physical matter moving through physical space and experienced as "time"; the *Awareness* held by *Self* that is restricted to an organic *Lifeform* or "*genetic vehicle*" in which it experiences causality in *beta-existence*.

beta (existence) : all manifestation in the "Physical Universe" (KI, in *Zuism*); the conditions of *Awareness* for the *Alpha-spirit* (*Self*) as a physical organic *Lifeform* or "*genetic vehicle*" in which it experiences causality in the *Physical Universe*.

charge : to fill or furnish with a quality; to supply with energy; to lay a command upon; in *Systemology*—to imbue with intention; to overspread with emotion; personal energy stores and significances entwined as fragmentation in mental images, reactive-response encoding and intellectual (and/or) programmed beliefs.

channel : a specific stream, course, current, direction or route; to form or cut a groove or ridge or otherwise guide along a specific course; a direct path; an artificial aqueduct created to connect two water bodies or water or make travel possible.

circuit : a circular path or loop; a closed-path within a system that allows a flow; a pattern or action or wave movement that follows a specific route or potential path only; in *Systemology*, "*communication processing*" pertaining to a specific *flow* of energy or information along a channel; "*feedback loop.*"

communication : successful transmission of information, data, energy (&tc.) along a message line, with a reception of feedback; an energetic flow of intention to cause an effect (or duplication) at a distance; the personal energy moved or acted upon by will or else 'selective directed attention'; the 'messenger action' used to transmit and receive energy across a medium; also relay of energy, a message or signal—or even locating a personal POV (viewpoint) for the Self—along the *ZU-line.*

condense (condensation) : the transition of vapor to liquid; denoting a change in state to a more substantial or solid condition; leading to a more compact or solid form.

confront : to come around in front of; to be in the presence of; to stand in front of, or in the face of; to meet "face-to-face" or "face-up-to"; additionally, in *Systemology*, to fully tolerate or acceptably withstand an encounter with a particular manifestation without an automatic reactive response.

consideration : careful analytical reflection of all aspects; deliberation; determining the significance of a "thing" in relation to similarity or dissimilarity to other "things"; evaluation of facts and importance of certain facts; thorough examination of all aspects related to, or important for, making a decision; the analysis of consequences and estimation of significance when making decisions; also in *Systemology*, the *postulate* or *Alpha-Thought* that defines the state of *beingness* for what something "*is.*"

defragmentation : the *reparation* of wholeness; collecting all dispersed parts to reform an original whole; a process of removing "*fragmentation*" in data or knowledge to provide a clear understanding; applying techniques and processes that promote a *holistic* interconnected *alpha* state, favoring observational *Awareness* of continuity in all spiritual and physical systems; in *Systemology*, a "*Seeker*" achieving actualized "*Self-Honest Awareness*" is said to be in a basic state of *beta-defragmentation*, whereas *Alpha-defragmentation* is the rehabilitation of the *creative ability*, managing the *Spiritual Timeline* and the POV of *Self* as Alpha-Spirit (I-AM).

existence : the *state* or fact of *apparent manifestation*; the resulting combination of the Principles of Manifestation: consciousness, motion

117

and substance; continued *survival*; that which independently exists.

exterior : outside of; on the outside; in *System-ology*, we mean specifically the POV of *Self* that is *'outside of'* the *Human Condition,* free of the physical and mental trappings of the Physical Universe; a metahuman range of consideration; see also *'Zu-Vision'*.

external : a force coming from outside; inform-ation received from outside sources; in *System-ology*, the objective *'Physical Universe'* exist-ence, or *beta-existence*, that the Physical Body or *genetic vehicle* is essentially *anchored* to for its considerations of locational space-time as a dimension or POV.

fragmentation : breaking into parts and scatter-ing the pieces; the *fractioning* of wholeness or the *fracture* of a holistic interconnected *alpha* state, favoring observational *Awareness* of per-ceived connectivity between parts; *discontinu-ity*; separation of a totality into parts; in *Systemology*, a person outside of *Self-Honesty* is said to be operating from a *fragmented* state.

flow : movement across (or through) a channel (or conduit); a direction of active energetic mo-tion, typically distinguished as either an *in-flow*, *out-flow* or *cross-flow*.

genetic-vehicle : a physical *Life*-form; the physical (*beta*) body that is animated/controlled by the (*Alpha*) *Spirit* using a continuous *Spiritual Lifeline* (ZU); a physical (*beta*) organic receptacle and catalyst for the (*Alpha*) *Self* to operate "causes" and experience "effects" within the *Physical Universe*.

harmful-act : a counter-survival mode of behavior or action (esp. that causes harm to one of more *Spheres of Existence*)—or—an overtly aggressive (hostile and/or destructive) action against an individual or any other *Sphere of Existence*; in *Utilitarian Systemology*—a short-sighted (serves fewest/lowest *Spheres of Existence*) intentional overtly harmful action to resolve a perceived problem; a revision of the rule for standard *Utilitarianism* for Systemology to distinguish actions which provide the least benefit to the least number of *Spheres of Existence*, or else the greatest harm to the greatest number of *Spheres of Existence*; in *moral philosophy*—an action which can be experienced by few and/or which one would not be willing to experience for themselves (*theft, slander, rape, &tc*); an iniquity or iniquitous act.

hold-back : withheld communications (esp. actions) such as "*Hold-Outs*"; intentional (or automatic) withdrawal (as opposed to reach); Self-restraint (which may eventually be enforced or automated); not reaching, acting or expressing, when one should be; an ability that is now restrained (on automatic) due to inability to withhold it on Self-determinism alone.

hold-outs : in photography, the numerous snapshots/pictures withheld from the final display or professional presentation of the event; withheld communications; in Utilitarian Systemology— energetic withdrawal and communication breaks with a "*terminal*" and its *Sphere of Existence* as a result of a "*Harmful-Act*"; unspoken or undiscovered (hidden, covert) actions that an individual withholds communications of, fearing punishment or endangerment of *Self-preservation* (*First Sphere*); the act of hiding (or keeping hidden) the truth of a "*Harmful-Act*"; a refusal to communicate with a *Pilot*; also "*Hold-Back.*"

holistic : the examination of interconnected systems as encompassing something greater than the *sum* of their "parts."

Human Condition : a standard default state of Human experience that is generally accepted to be the extent of its potential identity (*beingness*) —currently treated as *Homo Sapiens Sapiens,* but which is scheduled for replacement by *Homo Novus* (the "New Human").

imagination : ability to create *mental imagery* in one's Personal Universe at will and change or alter it as desired; the ability to create, change and dissolve mental images on command or as an act of will; to create a mental image or have associated imagery displayed (or "conjured") in the mind that may or may not be treated as real (or memory recall) and may or may not accurately duplicate objective reality; to employ *creative abilities* of the Spirit that are independent of reality agreements with beta-existence.

imprint : to strongly impress, stamp, mark (or outline) onto a softer 'impressible' substance; to mark with pressure onto a surface; in *Systemology,* used to indicate permanent Reality impressions marked by frequencies, energies or interactions experienced during periods of emotional distress, pain, unconsciousness, loss, enforcement, or something antagonistic to physical (personal) survival, all of which are are stored with other reactive response-mechanisms at lower-levels of *Awareness* as opposed to the active memory database and proactive processing center of the Mind; an experiential "memory-set" that may later resurface—be triggered or stimulated artificially—as Reality, of which similar responses will be engaged automatically; holographic-like imagery "stamped" onto consciousness as composed of energetic *facets* tied to the "snap-shot" of an experience.

imprinting incident : the first or original event

instance communicated and *emotionally encoded* onto an individual's "*Spiritual Timeline*" (recorded memory from all lifetimes), which formed a permanent impression that is later used to mechanistically treat future contact on that channel; the first or original occurrence of some particular *facet* or mental image related to a certain type of *encoded response*, such as pain and discomfort, losses and victimization, and even the acts that we have taken against others along the *Spiritual Timeline* of our existence that caused them to also be *Imprinted*.

intention : directed application of Will; to intend (have "in Mind") or signify (give "significance" to) for or toward a particular purpose; in *Systemology* (from the *Standard Model*)—the spiritual activity at WILL (5.0) directed by an *Alpha Spirit* (7.0); the application of WILL as "Cause" from a higher order of Alpha Thought and consideration (6.0).

interior : inside of; on the inside; in *Systemology*, we mean specifically the POV of *Self* that is fixed to the *'internal' Human Condition,* including the *Reactive Control Center* (RCC) and Mind-System or *Master Control Center* (MCC); within *beta-existence*.

internal : a force coming from inside; information received from inside sources; in *Systemology*, the objective experience of *beta-existence* associated with the Physical Body or *genetic vehicle* and its POV regarding sensation and perception; from inside the body; in the body.

invalidate : decrease the level or degree or *agreement* as Reality.

mental image : a subjectively experienced "picture" created and imagined into being by the Alpha-Spirit (or at lower levels, one of its automated mechanisms) that includes all perceptible *facets* of totally immersive scene, which may be forms originated by an individual, or a "facsimile-copy" ("snap-shot") of something seen or encountered; a duplication of wave-forms in one's Personal Universe as a "picture" that mirror an "external" Universe experience, such as an *Imprint*.

perception : internalized processing of data received by the *senses*; to become *Aware of* via the senses.

pilot : a professional steersman responsible for healthy functional operation of a ship toward a specific destination; in *Systemology*, an intensive trained individual qualified to specially apply *Systemology Processing* to assist other *Seekers* on the *Pathway*.

point-of-view (POV) : a point to view from; an opinion or attitude as expressed from a specific identity-phase; a specific standpoint or vantage-point; a definitive manner of consideration specific to an individual phase or identity; a place or position affording a specific view or vantage; circumstances and programming of an individual that is conducive to a particular response, consideration or belief-set (paradigm); a position (consideration) or place (location) that provides a specific view or perspective (subjective) on experience (of the objective).

postulate : to put forward as truth; to suggest or assume an existence *to be*; to state or affirm the existence of particular conditions; to provide a basis of reasoning and belief; a basic theory accepted as fact; in *Systemology*, Alpha-Thought —the top-most decisions or considerations made by the Alpha-Spirit regarding the "*is-ness*" (what things "are") about energy-matter and space-time.

presence : a quality of some thing (*energy/matter*) being "present" in space-time; personal orientation of *Self* as an *Awareness* (*POV*) located in present space-time (environment) and communicating with extant energy-matter.

processing command line (PCL) : a directed input; a specific command using highly selective language for *Systemology Processing*; a predetermined directive statement (cause) intended to focus concentrated attention (effect).

processing, systematic : the inner-workings or "through-put" result of systems; in *Systemology*, a method of applied spiritual technology used toward personal Self-Actualization; methods of selective directed attention, communicated language and associative imagery that increases personal control of the human condition.

realization : the clear perception of an understanding; a consideration or understanding on what is "actual"; to make "real" or give "reality" to so as to grant a property of "being-ness" or "being as it is"; the state or instance of coming to an *Awareness*; in *Systemology*, "gnosis" or true knowledge achieved during *systematic processing*; achievement of a new (or higher) cognition, true knowledge or perception of Self; a consideration of reality or assignment of meaning.

responsibility : the *ability* to *respond*; the extent of mobilizing *power* and *understanding* an individual maintains as *Awareness* to enact *change*; the proactive ability to *Self-direct* and make decisions independent of an outside authority.

Seeker : an individual on the *Pathway to Self-Honesty*; a practitioner of *Mardukite Systemology* or *Systemology Processing*, that is working toward *Spiritual Ascension*.

Self-actualization : bringing the full potential of the Human spirit into Reality; expressing full capabilities and creativeness of the *Alpha-Spirit*.

Self-determinism : the freedom to act, clear of external control or influence; the personal control of Will to direct intention.

Self-honesty : the basic or original *alpha* state of *being* and *knowing*; clear and present total *Awareness* of-and-as *Self*, in its most basic and true proactive expression of itself as *Spirit* or *I-AM*—free of artificial attachments, perceptive filters and other emotionally-reactive or mentally-conditioned programming imposed on the human condition by the systematized physical world; the ability to experience existence without judgment.

spiritual timeline : a continuous stream of moment-to-moment *Mental Images* (or a record of experiences) that defines the "past" of a spiritual being (or *Alpha-Spirit*) and which includes impressions (*imprints, &tc.*) from all life-incarnations and significant spiritual events the being has encountered; in Systemology, also "*backtrack*."

Spheres of Existence : a series of *eight* concentric circles, rings or spheres (each larger than the former) that is overlaid onto the Standard Model of Beta-Existence to demonstrate the dynamic systems of existence extending out from the POV of Self (often as a "body") at the *First Sphere*; these are given in the basic eightfold systems as: *Self, Home/Family, Groups, Humanity, Life on Earth, Physical Universe, Spiritual Universe* and *Infinity-Divinity.*

Systemology : a modern tradition of applied religious philosophy and spiritual technology based on *Arcane Tablets* (in combination with "*general systemology*" and "*games theory*") developed in the New Age underground by Joshua Free in 2011 as an advanced futurist extension of the *Mardukite Research Org.*

terminal (node) : a point, end, or mass, on a line; a connection point for closing an electric circuit, such as a post on a battery terminating at each end of its own systematic function; a point of connectivity with other points; in systems, a contact point of interaction; a point of interaction with other points.

turbulence : a quality or state of distortion or disturbance that creates irregularity of a flow or pattern; the quality or state of aberration on a line (such as ragged edges) or the emotional "turbulent feelings" attached to a particular flow or terminal node; a violent, haphazard or disharmonious commotion (such as in the ebb of gusts and lulls of wind action).

validation : a reinforcement of agreements or considerations as being "real."

viewpoint : see *"point-of-view" (POV)*.

willingness : the state of conscious Self-determined ability and interest (directed attention) to *Be*, *Do* or *Have*; a Self-determined consideration to reach, face up to (*confront*) or manage some "mass" or energy; the extent to which an individual considers themselves able to participate, act or communicate along some line, to put attention or intention on the line, or to produce (create) an effect.

ZU : the ancient Sumerian cuneiform sign for the archaic verb—*"to know," "knowingness"* or *"awareness"*; in *Mardukite Zuism and Systemology*, the active energy/matter of the "Spiritual Universe" (AN) experienced as a *Lifeforce* or *consciousness* that imbues living forms extant in the "Physical Universe" (KI); *"Spiritual Life Energy"*; energy demonstrated by the WILL of an actualized *Alpha-Spirit* in the "Spiritual Universe" (AN), which impinges its *Awareness* into the Physical Universe (KI), animating/controlling *Life* for its experience of *beta-existence* along an individual Alpha-Spirit's personal *Identity-continuum*, called a *ZU-line*.

Zu-Line : a theoretical construct in *Mardukite Zuism and Systemology* demonstrating *Spiritual*

Life Energy (*ZU*) as a personal individual "continuum" of Awareness interacting with all Spheres of Existence on the Standard Model of Systemology; a spectrum of potential variations and interactions of a monistic continuum or singular *Spiritual Life Energy* demonstrated on the Standard Model; an energetic channel of potential POV and "locations" of Beingness, demonstrated in early Systemology materials as an individual Alpha-Spirit's personal *Identity- continuum*, potentially connecting *Awareness* of *Self* with "*Infinity*" simultaneous with all points considered in existence; a symbolic demonstration of the "*Life-line*" on which *Awareness (ZU)* extends from the direction of the "Spiritual Universe" (AN) in its true original *alpha state* through an entire possible range of activity resulting in its *beta state* and control of a *genetic-entity* occupying the *Physical Universe (KI).*

Zu-Vision : the true and basic (*Alpha*) Point-of-View (perspective, POV) maintained by *Self* as *Alpha-Spirit* outside boundaries or considerations of the *Human Condition* and *exterior* to beta-existence reality agreements with the Physical Universe; a POV of Self *as* "a unit of Spiritual Awareness" that exists independent of a "body" and entrapment in a *Human Condition*; "spirit vision" in its truest sense.

Collector's Edition Hardcover

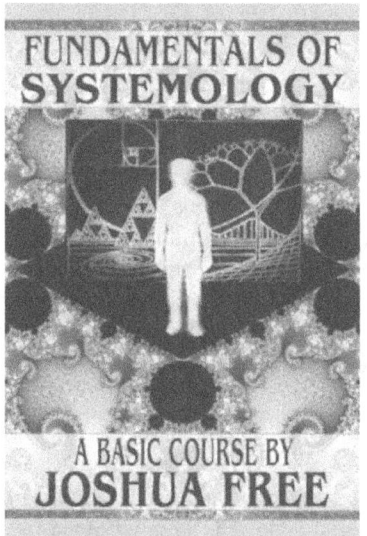

THE FUNDAMENTALS OF
SYSTEMOLOGY

A Basic Course developed by
Joshua Free

*collecting material of six lesson-booklets
together in one volume!*

"Being More Than Human"

"Realities in Agreement"

"Windows To Experience"

"Ancient Systemology"

"A History of Systemology"

"Systemology Processing"

All *six* lesson-booklets of the first official
Basic Course on Mardukite Systemology
are combined together in *one volume* as
"Fundamentals of Systemology."

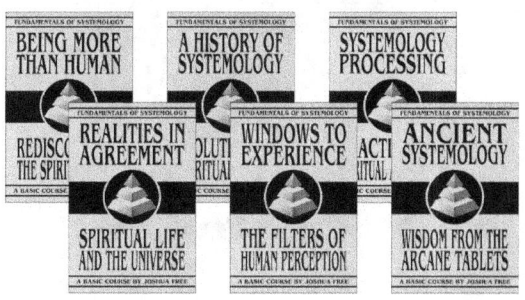

Lesson booklets are also available individually!

Collector's Edition Hardcover

THE PATHWAY TO
ASCENSION

The Systemology
Professional Course by
Joshua Free

All sixteen lessons available in two volumes!

"Increasing Awareness"

"Thought & Emotion"

"Clear Communication"

"Handling Humanity"

"Free Your Spirit"

"Escaping Spirit-Traps"

"Eliminating Barriers"

"Conquest of Illusion"

...and more!

All *sixteen* lesson-booklets of the newest
Professional Course on Mardukite Systemology
are combined together in *two volumes* as
"The Pathway to Ascension."

Lesson booklets are also available individually!

THE SYSTEM

Seekers and students of the *Professional Course* and *Advanced Training Course* will also be interested in the original *Systemology Core Research Series.* These *8* volumes are a complete chronological record of *Mardukite NexGen New Thought* developments published by the *Systemology Society* from 2019 through 2023.

The Systemology Core series begins with the first professional publication released when our *Mardukite Systemology* emerged from the underground in 2019, with: *"The Tablets of Destiny Revelation."*

OLOGY CORE

The Tablets of Destiny Revelation:
*How Long-Lost Anunnaki Wisdom
Can Change the Fate of Humanity*

Crystal Clear: *Handbook for Seekers*

Metahuman Destinations (2 *volumes*)

Imaginomicon:
Approaching Gateways to Higher Universes

Way of the Wizard: *Utilitarian Systemology*

Systemology-180: *Fast-Track to Ascension*

Systemology Backtrack:
Reclaiming Spiritual Power & Past-Life Memory

PUBLISHED BY THE **JOSHUA FREE** IMPRINT REPRESENTING

The Mardukite Academy of Systemology

mardukite.com

CONQUEST OF
ILLUSION

POCKET EDITION

Published from
Mardukite Borsippa HQ, San Luis Valley, Colorado
Mardukite Academy & Systemology Society
for spiritual or educational purposes only

CONQUEST
OF ILLUSION

Systemology
Professional Course
Booklet #8

Developed by Joshua Free
for the Systemology Society

THE JOSHUA FREE IMPRINT
JFI PUBLICATIONS

Pocket Paperback Edition — *December 2023*

mardukite.com

Chart Your Flight For Ascension...
Then Let Your Spirit Fly!

Unlock your ultimate spiritual potential by removing barriers to your true native state.

Learn how to easily attain Self-actualization and help to actualize others along the way.

A greater appreciation and understanding of *Spiritual Life* and *Existence* awaits you. Expand your reach to achieve your dreams.

Each 'Professional Course' lesson-booklet offers simple exercises and techniques that directly apply the philosophy of Systemology, assisting to increase your true knowingness, improve your capabilities in this life, and even decide what you will do in your next.

At the Mardukite Academy of Systemology, the 'Professional Course' lessons in this series are presented to Seeker's that have already completed the 'Basic Course', previously released as six lesson-booklets, or the six-in-one single volume edition "Fundamentals of Systemology."

This all new presentation of the Systemology 'Pathway-to-Ascension' takes Seekers and continuing students from "Zero" to "Infinity" at lightning-fast speeds!

Discover Who You Really Are...
Because You Were Never Human

<u>Fundamentals of Systemology</u>
Basic Course Lesson Booklet Series

#1 – *Being More Than Human*
#2 – *Realities In Agreement*
#3 – *Windows To Experience*
#4 – *Ancient Systemology*
#5 – *A History of Systemology*
#6 – *Systemology Processing*

<u>The Pathway to Ascension</u>
Professional Course Lesson Booklet Series

#1 – *Increasing Awareness*
#2 – *Thought & Emotion*
#3 – *Clear Communication*
#4 – *Handling Humanity*
#5 – *Free Your Spirit*
#6 – *Escaping Spirit-Traps*
#7 – *Eliminating Barriers*
#8 – *Conquest of Illusion*
#9 – *Confronting the Past*

...more titles in this series coming soon!

TABLET OF CONTENTS

PROFESSIONAL
COURSE
INTRODUCTION

WELCOME, SEEKER!
LET'S CHART YOUR JOURNEY
ON THE PATHWAY

Systemology is a "holistic" approach to understanding the human experience. It is not actually a singular "subject" in itself, but rather, a new way in which to view the many subjects of *Life* and all *Existence.*

This is a professional course in *Systemology*—specifically, how to *apply* the spiritual philosophy of *Mardukite Systemology* as a personal *"Pathway"* to Ascension. Our *Systemology* is a new approach to *"Self-Actualization."* It is completely relevant for the modern age and the future; and quite different from any previous similar attempts, or other traditions, you might find. What's more: it is applicable to anyone with any background.

This *"Professional Course"* series of lessons (booklets) immediately follows the material given in the *"Basic Course"* series—available as six separate pocket-sized booklets, or in a single hardcover volume titled: *"Fundamentals of Systemology: A New Thought For The 21st Century."*

This is a *new* presentation of *Systemology*, emphasizing the application of our philosophy for those *Seekers* that are *"Flying-Solo"*—or else working through their studies and exercises as solitary practitioners. This is a new innovation for *Systemology*. Aside from the book *"Crystal Clear,"* all of our former advanced courses have placed a focus on *"Traditional Piloting"*—where experienced practitioners assist *Seekers* in *"processing."*

To receive the greatest benefit from this study: it is expected that a *Seeker* will already be familiar with the fundamental concepts and terminology (previously re-

layed in the *Basic Course*) before using lessons from the *Professional Course*. This will allow us to cover the extensive territory of the *Pathway* much more quickly. However, for reference, a basic *"glossary"* of vocabulary used in this lesson is provided in the *"appendix."*

A NEW VIEW OF THE HUMAN SPIRIT

Systemology is not a religion and does not require any type of *faith*. It is, however, built upon a "spiritual" premise—and as such is an "applied spiritual philosophy." It is based on ancient teachings that we are *Spiritual Beings* essentially "wearing" bodies like clothes—or using them as "vehicles." Yet our true native nature is not *physical*, but beyond this existence; and we can certainly operate a "body" from *outside* of it.

We are **all** *Spiritual Beings*—each of us a *unit* of *Spiritual Awareness*—that have experienced a very long *Spiritual Timeline* of existence. Although we might be particularly attached to the familiar "physical shells" associated with *this* lifetime, our true "*Spiritual Lifetime*" is seemingly *eternal*. We have been many things before *Human*, and we go onward as a *Spiritual Being* after our "*genetic vehicle*" of *this* incarnation perishes.

While a "spiritual" view of the *Human Condition* may not seem unique to our philosophy, just how often is the concept treated *systematically*? For that matter: just how many people, supposedly raised to this or that religion, or professing to believe one thing or another, actually live their lives as though they are *Spirits*?

As *Spiritual Beings* of immortal existence and infinite potential, we are not simply the "*creations*" of an even greater *Being-*

ness; we are, in fact, an integral part of that *"creative force"* which permeates all existence.

Our basic nature is to be a *"creative being"*—our highest goals are *"to create."* And as such a being—which we refer to as an *Alpha-Spirit* in *Systemology*—we have run into some difficulties along the course of our *Spiritual Timeline* and found ourselves trapped within material *Universes* of our own collaborative *creation*.

Since we did not start out our existence in a trapped condition, it is correct to say that we have *"fallen"* from our native *"godlike"* states. It did not happen all at one, but progressively and systematically. We know our "troubles" have resulted from accumulated "barriers" and "blockages"—or *fragmentation*—during our vast experiences as *Spiritual Beings*. They are not because we lack something; but because of what's been added.

In *Systemology*, we systematically examine those routes by which we must have descended to reach our present condition, then reverse the direction of travel and chart a personal *"Pathway to Ascension."* Of course, the exact "details" of the *Spiritual Timeline* will be different for each individual *Seeker*. However, we have been able to systematically chart our *Pathway* based on common patterns of *Human fragmentation*.

In the most basic terms: the *fragmentation* that defines our "downward spiral" consists of decisions or considerations where we deny our true nature. This includes those decisions to *"withdraw"* rather than *"reach"*; where we choose to *not-know* rather than *know*; to *not-communicate* rather than *communicate*; and ultimately, to take *no-responsibility* for being a *creative-cause*, and therefore succumb to being an *effect*.

But there is *hope!* And much more im-
portantly: there is an effectively workable
way out of the mazes and traps of our existence. If you are reading this now, you
have already begun to gather your tools
and build up the *"horsepower"* necessary
to break the gravity holding your *Spiritual Beingness* to the *Human Condition*.

STUDYING THE
PROFESSIONAL COURSE

Most *Seekers* study and practice *Systemology* at-a-distance and independent of the
"Mardukite Academy" or any "Mas-
ter-level" mentors trained therein. This
means that the *books* (and to a lesser degree, the *internet*) are the only means of
direct contact a *Seeker* maintains with the
"Systemology Society" during their studies. A continuing *Seeker* from the *"Basic
Course"* will be familiar with the style of
study found in *this* course.

Misunderstood words are the most common reason an individual abandons studying a subject. When a misunderstanding occurs, *Awareness* declines. These misunderstandings start to "stack up" after the first occurrence, and as a result, the level of interest and attention will also decline. This is how a "confusion" develops; and the individual will get "bored" with the subject, feel tired, and unable to concentrate.

One solution is to return to the part of the material that was still interesting and enjoyable to read. When scanning around that area of text, there is likely to be a new word (or new specific use of a familiar word) that is unclear, but was passed by unnoticed. All *Systemology* books include their own *glossary*. Using this *glossary* and a high-quality dictionary will help resolve this misunderstanding once it is located.

An effective education of any subject is taught on a *gradient*. This is what is intended by presenting the study of something as "*grades*." Rather than treating a subject as one total mass, true learning is achieved by increasing one's understanding with a *gradual* increase upward. The *ascent* to a mountaintop is not successfully achieved in one leap, but by targeting and reaching specific checkpoints along the way.

This *Professional Course* consists of a series of lessons (booklets) that gradually increase a *Seeker's* ability to understand and apply the practices and techniques of *Systemology* as a complete "*Pathway to Ascension*." It is an appropriate study for continuing *Seekers* (from the *Basic Course*), but also "advanced" *Systemologists*.

Each lesson (booklet) of the *Professional Course* applies *Systemology* to a particular subject (or focus). It is best if the entire

course can be studied and applied in sequential order. These lessons also employ a style of practice or technique called "*Systematic Processing.*" An introduction to applying this methodology is provided in the final lesson (booklet) of the *Basic Course*—or in the "*Fundamentals of Systemology*" volume.

To study the *Professional Course* just like a student at the Academy: a *Seeker* reads through all instructional material and applies each exercise (or "*process*") presented in the text to the extent they comfortably can, before continuing on to the next lesson (booklet).

When first starting on the *Pathway* as a *Solo* practitioner, without the aid of an experienced *Pilot*, a *Seeker* shouldn't "push too hard" or allow themselves to get too "stuck" on any one area (lesson) or *process*. It is not expected that any one area will be completely handled when first in-

troduced. For optimum results, it is expected that a serious *Seeker* will make more than one "pass" through the entire *Professional Course.*

The *Professional Course* is not altogether different from other forms of practical or technical education: where the instruction and exercises are delivered to a completion, and then a student further increases their abilities, strength and skill-level by applying additional practice throughout their life. Therefore, a student should not concern themselves with perfectly mastering each step (or lesson) before progressing forward.

Additional passes through the material are likely to result in different *"realizations"* (an increased *level of understanding*) than a previous time. New "layers" of *Knowingness* may now be accessible during a *process* that may not have been before. It is important to avoid invalidating

the progress you've made just because one area is not completely handled right away, or if a certain *process* seems too difficult on the first pass.

CHARTING A COURSE ON THE PATHWAY

Although we can communicate a systematic structure to *fragmentation*, the personal journey experienced along the *Pathway* will be different for each *Seeker*. For example, certain areas will seem more "*turbulent*" or difficult for one *Seeker* than another. We tend to say that these areas have more "*charge*" on them—or that they are more "*heavily charged*." It is best to handle such areas when you are already feeling "good" and not in a situation (or condition) where that specific area is consistently being "*triggered*" or "*restimulated*."

As an applied philosophy, *Systemology* "theory" can be easily utilized in the "laboratory" of the "world-at-large" in everyday life. This is implied within the basic instruction of each lesson. Unlike other "sciences" that conduct experiments by making a change to some "objective variable" *out there* and waiting to see an effect, our focus is the individual (or *Observer*) themselves, and how *they* affect the *"Reality"* perceived.

In addition to applying *Systemology* "New Thought" to everyday life, our philosophy is applied by using specific exercises and systematic techniques. These *"processes"* provide the most stable personal gain (and *realizations*) for each area; but only when actually applied with a *Seeker's* full *"presence"* and *Awareness*.

This *Professional Course* is designed so that it may be easily read and studied with little concern for what "dangers"

23

these teachings—or *processing*—might unleash. However, there are still some guidelines that pertain to the "best-uses" of these course lessons, particularly if a *Seeker* intends for stable development.

Skipping over too much material/*processing* in early lessons may make attempts to understand (or apply) later lessons more difficult. However, once the complete *Professional Course* is worked through at least once in its entirety, specific areas can then be later returned to and treated with a greater sense of *Awareness* and *"presence"* than before. Of course, in *"Traditional Piloting,"* the rate of processing is monitored by an experienced practitioner; but in *"Solo-Processing,"* a *Seeker* must regulate their own progress on the *Pathway*.

Applying a systematic technique is called *"running a process."* The *processes* are designed with very simple instructions or

"*command-lines*." To *run* a *processing command-line*, a *Seeker* may be assisted by the communication of that *line* from a "*Co-Pilot*" (as in "*Traditional Piloting*"). But even then, a *Seeker* must still personally "input" the *command* as *Self*. For this reason —and quite thankfully— *Solo-Processing* is possible.

TAKING FLIGHT ON THE PATHWAY

Processing Techniques are intended to treat the *Spiritual Being* or *Alpha-Spirit*; the individual themselves. It is applied by the *Alpha-Spirit*—then *Self-directed* to the "Mind-System" or even a "body" (*genetic-vehicle*), both of which are "constructs" that the *Alpha-Spirit* (*Self*, or the "I-AM" *Awareness unit*) operates, but neither of which is actually *Self*. *Fragmentation* causes *Humans* to falsely identify *Self as* the "*Mind*" or even a "*Body*."

25

The *Professional Course* lessons (booklets) are designed for the *Beginning Seeker* in mind—one that may have an understanding of theory, but with little experience in practice. That being said: each of these lessons may be used toward total *Beta-Defragmentation* within a specific area. There are also more *processes* given for each subject than may be necessary to achieve an *ultimate end-point realization* on that entire area.

Some *processes* can be treated quite lightly at first; others may require a bit of working at in order to get *"running"* well. It is important to set aside a period of time when you can be dedicated to your studies and *processing.* This period of time is referred to as a *"processing session."* The reason for this, is that when a *process* does start *running* well, it is important to be able to complete it to a satisfactory *"end-point."*

The purpose of *systematic processing* is to be able to *really* "look" at things and even determine the *considerations* we have made—or attitudes we have decided—about *Reality* as a result of those experiences. It doesn't do us much good to simply "glance"—or to *restimulate* something uncomfortable and then quickly *withdraw* from it once again, leaving more of our *attention* yet again behind and held fixedly on it.

Generally speaking, a *Seeker* continues to *run* a *process* so long as something is "happening"—which is to say, the *process* is still producing a change. Usually this is evident by the type of "answers" that a *command-line* helps a *Seeker* originate from the database of their own *Mind-System*. The *command-lines* do not "do" anything on their own. They assist a *Seeker* to direct their own attention toward increasing *Awareness*.

Of course, a *Seeker* may also cease to generate new "data" from a *process* without reaching an *"ultimate" realization* as an *"end-point."* It is possible that additional "layers" (or even other "areas") require handling before anything "deeper" is accessible. If this is the case, end the *process*. But, if a *Seeker* is *withdrawing* from something uncomfortable that was incited or stirred up, then a *process* is *run* until they feel "good" about it.

In case the thought of encountering *"turbulence"* is a concern: the techniques given as *"Opening Procedures"* of a *Formal Session* (in the *Basic Course*), and those found in the earliest lessons of the *Professional Course*, are quite useful when applied as "safety nets" for maintaining *Awareness* and *presence*, even when *Flying-Solo*.

One of the benefits to *Flying-Solo* is that *processing* is entirely *Self-determined*. This

already provides a certain built-in "safe-ty" for a practitioner. Anything you *res-timulate* by *Self-determinism* is *your thing.* It is not incited by external *other-de-termined* influences (or other "source-points" in existence) that make you an *ef-fect*. It can be more easily handled in *pro-cessing*—or you can simply let things "cool down" and come back to it again.

While it may seem "mysterious" to be-ginners, a *Seeker* gets a sense for knowing how long to *run* a *process* only with prac-tice. Once you have spent some time ac-tually applying the *Professional Course*, there are many aspects that become "second nature" because they are, in fact, a part of our true original nature. All we have done is *"reverse engineer"* the routes of *creation* and *consideration* that are already *our own.*

LESSON EIGHT:
CONQUEST
OF ILLUSION

PERSONAL INTEGRITY

Our practice of *Systemology* toward *Ascension* is effective for the simple fact that: at the core, in our most basic state, the *Alpha-Spirit* is actually quite "righteous" and "good." This is what allows us to rehabilitate *abilities* and restore the level of *Awareness*. Nothing is being "added" to *Self* on the *Pathway*; it is the "additives" that are being "removed," and in doing so, removing the *barriers* and *blockages* of our true state.

We have already treated the preliminaries of "*Eliminating Barriers*" in our previous lesson (booklet). In this one, we continue further in this area to complete the necessary *systematic processing* for *Systemology Level-3*. Much of the material found in this lesson (booklet) is based on a book found in our *Systemology Core*, titled: "*The Way of the Wizard*."

At the inception of *Shared-Game Universes*, *Alpha-Spirits* went to great lengths to "trick" and "deceive" one another. This is because, during our early experiences as *god-like* beings—before we considered our *Self* to be attached to any kind of *"body"* that could be harmed—"deception" and "trickery" is about all that you could really do against another *god-like* being.

"Illusions" were originally created for fun and entertainment—similar to going to the "movies" or attending a "stage magic" show. Remember that, at basic, we as *Alpha-Spirits*, have a uniquely strong fondness for *"games."* But later on, more recently on the *Backtrack* of our *Spiritual Existence*, things became more serious as these "illusions" started to be used as a means of *entrapping* and *enslaving* each other.

This is not an easy area for many to handle or *process*. As such, many *Seekers*

that have started upon the *Pathway* often fall by the wayside, never progressing beyond this *processing level*. It is a lot to *confront* for some *Seekers*, which is why we only earn success with these areas after first completing the work provided in the previous lessons (booklets) of this *Professional Course*.

"CONFUSION" AND "FALSEHOOD"

It is sometimes quite challenging to differentiate between *truth* and *falsehood*, or to effectively *dispel illusion*. We have all had a lot of experience in mastering these skills. *Trickery* and *illusion* is also used to *conceal* the true native state that is available to us as *Alpha-Spirits*.

The *fragmentation* that stands as a *barrier* to the highest *realizations* of ourselves is almost entirely composed of *illusion* and *falsehood*. Our experience on the *Backtrack*,

in this lifetime and others, has afforded us a great bit of *fragmentation* concerning all sides of this area—what has been done to us and what we have done to others—and also what we have observed with others handling others.

Some of what would appear to be *"basic processing"* in this lesson is really intended to simply get a *Seeker* to actually recognize the facets associated with these various areas that have contributed to holding them back from the full *realization* of *Self*, in *Self-Honesty*, free of *fragmentation*, *compulsion* and *inhibition*.

When an individual *"Knows,"* they are not susceptible to *"falsehood."* Only after an *Alpha-Spirit* agrees to *"Not-Know"* (in order to have a *game*) will they fall prey to *trickery* and *deception*. One of the ways in which an *Alpha-Spirit* might be fooled, is through *misdirection* of *attention*— which is to say *"distraction."* It is this mechanism that allows a "stage magic-

ian" to fool an audience—and concealing what is *really* going on.

There is also the matter of *"confusion."* When one is in a state of *"confusion,"* they are quite likely to reinforce the solidity of *fragmentation* in their lives by reaching for the wrong piece of "data" in which to stabilize or orient themselves. States of *"confusion"* are so undesirable that an individual will grab a hold of anything that might bring resolution to the situation without fully analyzing and reviewing the content. And this is one way in which a person might be misled or manipulated to agree with *"false data."*

One of the most basic ways an individual overcomes *illusion* and *falsehood* is by *recognizing* it *"As-It-Is."* This becomes increasingly simpler to do as a *Seeker* elevates their level of *Actualized Awareness.* At high levels of personal application, *Awareness* is sufficient enough to unravel and disperse *fragmentation* "on

sight"—but only if *actually* "seen" *As-It-Is*, and not some false alteration of whatever "*It*" *is*.

The following *basic processes* employ the *"Analytical Recall"* technique described in former lessons. Their function is to help *realize* the type of areas we want to *resurface*, or bring into view, for *Systemology Level-3*.

Falsehood—Trickery/Fighting

1. *"Recall a time when you tricked someone into fighting."*

2. *"Recall a time when someone tricked you into fighting."*

3. *"Recall a time when someone tricked others into fighting."*

Falsehood—Distraction/Attention

1. *"Recall a time when you intentionally shifted someone's attention."*

2. *"Recall a time when someone intentionally shifted your attention."*

3. *"Recall a time when someone intentionally shifted another's attention."*

Falsehood — Confusion

1. *"Recall a time when you confused someone."*
2. *"Recall a time when someone confused you."*
3. *"Recall a time when someone confused others."*

As an additional exercise in identifying the *ideas* that we have used to resolve or reduce *confusion*, consider the following *process*:

A1. *"Recall a confusion."*
A2. *"What 'idea' resolved or reduced that confusion?"*

DEFRAGMENTING "FALSEHOOD"

There are always people in our societies that "instigate" or propagate *confusion, falsehood* and *suppression*. This is not unique to only life here on this planet. There are innumerable times in history when *conflict* or *confusion* was encouraged for someone's personal gain or to eliminate an opponent. In many ways this is an inherent part of *games* that involve "*players*" who perceive themselves as in "competition" with each other.

Information is easily mishandled—or *miscommunicated*. Whether intentionally given or otherwise, such *misinformation* or *false-data* is inherently *fragmentation*. It contributes to our having a false *perception* of our environment, and subsequently our making inaccurate evaluations when participating—*acting* and *doing* things—in existence. This *fragment-*

ation reduces our *Awareness* and the clarity of our memory.

One of the ways in which *falsehood* is spread, is by *"Passing the Buck."* We mean when *"blame"* is misplaced onto some individual, family, group, or society—race, country, &tc. This is a *misdirection* of *attention* (*Awareness*) from a "true source" to a "false source" (thereby disguising the *real* origination of an action).

Another commonly used tactic is to *misdirect* or *"shift"* the data about the date/timing of an event—replacing actual data with invented data. This not only obscures the facts, but can also either *"diminish"* or *"exaggerate"* the *significance* of the data—such as representing *events* as being "longer ago" than they actually are, &tc.

Sometimes efforts to *"shift significance"* of facts are more direct. For example, someone might overtly (visibly or obviously) "downplay" or "exaggerate" the

perceived importance (*significance*) of some data for their own covert (hidden) purposes or gains. This also occurs when someone acts to *embarrass, belittle* or *shame* an individual. Such *"suppressive"* individuals tend to hinder expressions of *creativity* and *ability*.

The following *processes* employ *"Analytical Recall"* to assist a *Seeker* in *recognizing* and *identifying* the presence of *"misdirection"* and *"manipulation"* in their own lives (and in memory, or on the *Backtrack*). *Processes* like these *may* lead to some new *end-realization*; but more often, directly *confronting* the *imprinted* memory of such areas of *fragmentation* will result in *relief/release* and increased *Awareness*.

Falsehood—Shifting Blame

1. *"Recall a time when you tried to shift blame onto another."*

2. *"Recall a time when someone tried to shift blame onto you."*

3. *"Recall a time when someone tried to shift blame onto another."*

Falsehood—Shifting Time

1. *"Recall misleading someone about the time when something occurred."*

2. *"Recall someone misleading you about the time when something occurred."*

3. *"Recall someone misleading others about the time when something occurred."*

Falsehood—Shifting Significance

1A. *"Recall a time when you exaggerated the importance of something."*

1B. *"Recall a time when you downplayed the importance of something."*

2A. *"Recall a time when someone else exaggerated the importance of something."*

2B. *"Recall a time when someone else downplayed the importance of something."*

Falsehood—Embarrassment/Shame

1. *"Recall a time when you made another embarrassed."*

2. *"Recall a time when someone made you embarrassed."*

3. *"Recall a time when someone made another embarrassed."*

Falsehood — Accusations

1. *"Recall a time when you falsely accused someone."*

2. *"Recall a time when someone falsely accused you."*

3. *"Recall a time when someone falsely accused another (or others)."*

Falsehood — Encouraged Conflict

A. *"Spot a time when you were told that someone (or something) was bad."*

B. *"Identify the person that told you that."*

C. *"Did that person have personal interests invested? How so?"*

Falsehood — True/False

A. *"Spot something you were told that you found out to be true."*

B. *"Spot something you were told that you found out to be false."*

Falsehood—Manipulation

1. *"How have you misled (or manipulated) another?"*

2. *"How has another misled (or manipulated) you?"*

3. *"How has another misled (or manipulated) others?"*

HANDLING "SUPPRESSION"

As a *Seeker* progresses along the *Pathway*, more and more of the "hiccups" and "up-sets" of the *Human Condition*—and experience of life in general—are able to be *confronted "As-It-Is"* (how things actually are).

Most of us have encountered at least one individual in our present lifetime that continually "acts" toward *creating* chall-

45

enges and difficulties for you personally. Some individuals apply this *effort* to larger groups of people, or even society as a whole. Those maintaining "higher" levels of *Actualized Awareness* are generally in a better position to handle such people directly, or at least the situations that they are *creating*.

A highly *Self-Actualized* individual doesn't succumb to suppression. It is possible, sometimes, to "win an enemy over" (getting them to accept/agree with your "side" or *reality*). If you can maintain your own "integrity" or "position" strongly or long enough, sometimes it is sufficient to "drive them off," or simply "wait them out" until the matter is dropped. But, this all requires being free of *automatic reactive-responses*.

There are also those unexpected or intense situations when an individual quickly becomes *overwhelmed*—the sense that one has become *too much* the *effect* of

the environment (or external source). The best course of action in this case is to remove yourself from the overwhelming influence and "catch your breath" in a safe position. This isn't a *withdrawal*, when ultimately, the situation will still have to be *confronted "As-It-Is."*

One reason why these persons and situations are so challenging for many individuals to handle, is because, quite often: the "present occurrence" *restimulates* much older (and longer) *"chains of fragmentation"* —stirring up *turbulence* from similar situations in the past that were left unresolved (*not-confronted*). This is what influences our succumbing to external "pressures."

Enslavement and *Domination* are *games* as old as the *Backtrack* itself. In fact, there are some individuals that carry *"fragmented purposes"* with them that are left over from *old games* (often from "past lives") they still have a lot of their *Awareness*

"stuck" on. They are still "playing" or "acting" in *this life* and *this game*, the *"roles"* or *"goals"* that they clung to long ago. That creates difficulties for others also playing on *this field*.

While it is easy to identify the more obvious situations we have encountered, it is the *"covert attacks"* and *"passive-aggressive" efforts* to *dominate* or *invalidate* us, that many *Seekers* are unprepared to handle in life. The most dangerous of our supposed "opponents" are those that specifically attempt to *"suppress"* our progress, gains, creative ability, and of course, advancement on the *Pathway-to-Ascension*.

A *personality* or *player* that is a *suppressive-type* will consistently try to *invalidate*—or "make less of"—you. Their general aim for *control* is to *"stop action."* Encounters with such types tend to leave us feeling "depressed" or "hopeless"—and yet they may also attempt to make us, in some way, "dependent" on them.

It is senseless to try to avoid all encounters with *domination* and *competition* in this *Universe*. It is an inherent part of the "*roles*" and "*goals*" perceived as part of the *game*; but many players are perceiving and operating with "*fragmented purposes*" —and they do not improve our experience of the *Game of Life* in any way.

The most desirable position (or solution) is to simply be in such "good condition" (as an *Actualized Seeker*) that these "external" (*other-determined*) *efforts* do not have enough "impact" to *invalidate* you— that your level of *Awareness* "exceeds" the degree or level of *energy* or *force* being "thrown at" you, and it may be essentially dissolved "*As-It-Is*." There is no reason to react or engage with further *energy* or *force*, which are of a "lower" order or condition of *existence* and *creation* than a *Self-Actualized Alpha-Spirit* is capable of.

DEFRAGMENTING "SUPPRESSION"

As mentioned above, most *suppressive control* is aimed at *"stopping motion"* (or action). While there are ways of being *constructively critical*, most *criticism* is intended to reduce or "make nothing" of another's *efforts* or *creations*. The following *basic processes* will help in identifying these *occurrences*. [We employ the word *"spot"* in these PCL to more accurately apply this *processing* to the full *Backtrack*.]

Suppression—Stops

1. *"Spot a time when you stopped someone."*

2. *"Spot a time when someone stopped you."*

3. *"Spot a time when someone stopped another (or others)."*

0. *"Spot a time when you stopped yourself."*

Suppression—Criticism

1. *"Spot a time when you criticized someone."*

2. *"Spot a time when someone criticized you."*

3. *"Spot a time when someone criticized another (or others)."*

0. *"Spot a time when you criticized yourself."*

Suppression—Invalidation

1. *"Spot a time when you 'made nothing' of someone."*

2. *"Spot a time when someone 'made nothing' of you."*

3. *"Spot a time when someone 'made nothing' of another (or others)."*

0. *"Spot a time when you 'made nothing' of yourself."*

It is not uncommon to find that encounters with a very *"suppressive-type"* during childhood can remain influential later on in life—even when that individual is no longer present. But that is how *imprints* work. When *Solo-Processing* the following exercise, use your *notebook* or *Flight-log* to

record the data from each PCL-question. List multiple answers (if necessary) to make sure you have answered each fully.

A. *"Is there anyone around whom you seem to become 'sick' shortly after seeing them?"*

B. *"Is there anyone who is continuously critical of you?"*

C. *"Is there anyone who is often telling you how 'bad' other people are?"*

D. *"Is there anyone who continuously 'stops' you?"*

E. *"Is there anyone who continuously 'invalidates' you?"*

F. *"Is there anyone who often provides 'false' information?"*

G. *"Is there anyone who often 'makes nothing' of your efforts?"*

If you find yourself writing the same name on several lists, then *run* the following *processes* using that name as the *"terminal"* (blank space) in the PCL. If there

are multiple names that frequently appear, then *run* those names as *terminals* too (each as their own series of *processes*). There is no "judgment" applied here about someone else's *intentions* toward us. The very fact that their name shows up frequently on these "lists" is sufficient to indicate there is enough *charge* present (as *fragmentation*) to be *run* as *processing*.

The following series of *processes* begins with a familiar one (from previous lessons) regarding "*help*." The purpose is not to enforce actually helping someone, but to restore the free choice (that is not overridden by *fragmentation*). *Considerations* of "*help*" also assist in breaking down the *barriers* of negative reactive emotion so that a *Seeker* is better able to actually confront the source of *suppression* "As-It-Is."

Suppressive Terminal — Help

1. "*How could you help ---?*"
2. "*How could --- help you?*"

3A. *"How could --- help others?"*

3B. *"How could others help ---?"*

Suppressive Terminal—Problems

1A. *"What 'problem' have you been to ---?"*

1B. *"What have they done about that?"*

2A. *"What 'problem' has --- been to you?"*

2B. *"What have you done about that?"*

3A. *"What 'problem' has --- been to others?"*

3B. *"What have others done about that?"*

4A. *"What 'problem' have others been to ---?"*

4B. *"What have they done about that?"*

Suppressive Terminal—Hold-Outs

1. *"What haven't you said to ---?"*

2. *"What hasn't --- said to you?"*

3. *"What hasn't --- said to others?"*

Suppressive Terminal—Actions

1. *"What have you done to ---?"*

2. *"What has --- done to you?"*

3A. *"What has --- done to others?"*

3B. *"What have others done to ---?"*

Suppressive Terminal—Invalidation

1. *"How have you 'invalidated' ---?"*

2. *"How has --- 'invalidated' you?"*

3A. *"How has --- 'invalidated' others?"*

3B. *"How have others 'invalidated' ---?"*

Each of the next three *processes* contains six alternating PCL. They are *run* using *"Analytical Recall"* techniques—although in this case, there may sometimes not be any available answer for a certain question. Any *turbulence* or *resistance* attached may then be handled using what you learned about *factors* in *Lesson-7.*

Trouble Sources—Likingness Factor

1A. *"Is there a time when you rejected their affection (or attention)?"*

1B. *"Is there a time when they rejected your affection (or attention)?"*

2A. *"Is there a time when you insisted that they like you?"*

2B. *"Is there a time when they insisted that you like them?"*

3A. *"Is there a time when you did like them?"*

3B. *"Is there a time when they did like you?"*

Trouble Sources—Communication Factor

1A. *"Is there a time when you rejected their communication?"*

1B. *"Is there a time when they rejected your communication?"*

2A. *"Is there a time when you insisted that they listen to you?"*

2B. *"Is there a time when they insisted that you listen to them?"*

3A. *"Is there a time when you communicated well with them?"*

3B. *"Is there a time when they communicated well with you?"*

Trouble Sources — Agreement Factor

1A. *"Is there a time when you refused to agree with them?"*

1B. *"Is there a time when they refused to agree with you?"*

2A. *"Is there a time when you insisted that they agree with you?"*

2B. *"Is there a time when they insisted that you agree with them?"*

3A. *"Is there a time when you did agree with them?"*

3B. *"Is there a time when they did agree with you?"*

Trouble Sources — Handling

A. *"What could you confront about ---?"*

B. *"What action of --- could you be responsible for?"*

C. *"What about --- could you be at cause over?"*

"JUSTIFICATION" & "RESPONSIBILITY"

Although we have discussed *"justifica-tion"* and *"responsibility"* briefly in passing up to this point of the *Pathway*, it is here at the end of *Systemology Level-3* that they are handled more directly. Although these words may appear commonly used, for *systematic processing*, we are primarily concerned with automatic reactivity regarding *compulsive action* (or *compulsive reach*) and *avoidance of action* (or *reactive withdrawal*).

The concepts of *"reach"* and *"withdrawal"* are familiar to us (by this point of the *Professional Course*), but to this, we also add the *"willingness to be responsible."* And by this, we don't mean "being blamed for things." We are speaking of a much higher-level of *"responsibility"* —as in: *"willingness* to be *at cause* over things."

Whenever an individual does something that they consider wrong—whether intentionally or otherwise—there is an *automatic* tendency to attempt to *"justify"* these actions. We do this when *communicating* about such things to others (assuming we don't *hold-out* on the information altogether)—but we also communicate these *"justifications"* to ourselves, and those *considerations* continue to affect us in the future.

In systematic terms: *justification* is a mishandling of *imprinting* or *"charge"* accumulated from an event (and possibly connected like a "chain" to similar events occurring earlier on the *Backtrack*). It strengthens the influence of *fragmentation*, because the "experiential data" is being *altered* rather than *confronted* "As-It-Is"—meaning: *reality* is being presented or perceived as *other than* it *actually is*; the worldview is distorted.

Maintaining (or *compulsively creating*) jus-

tifications" or *"falsehoods"* conflicts with the state of *Self-Honesty* sought as a means of *Ascension*. Maintaining any kind of *"false data"* or *fragmented thought* also leads an individual toward *fragmented actions* that are then used to support (or prove) the *justifications*.

The following *processes* are best *run* as "listing exercises," so be sure to have your *notebook* or *Flight-log* handy. They assist in later bringing a *primary "justification consideration"* into view (which the *Seeker* is operating with the most during this lifetime)—which is the *end-point* of *Systemology Level-3*.

Justification—General

1A. *"What have you done to another?"*

1B. *"How did you justify that?"*

2A. *"What has another done to you?"*

2B. *"How have they justified that?"*

3A. *"What has someone done to others?"*

3B. *"How have they justified that?"*

Justification—Excuses

A1. *"What do you often use as an excuse?"*

A2. *"What do others often use as an excuse?"*

B1. *"How could you survive without excuses?"*

B2. *"How could others survive without excuses?"*

Willingness—Improvement

1. *"What are you willing to improve?"*

2. *"What are you willing to allow others to improve?"*

3A. *"What would someone be willing to have you improve?"*

3B. *"What would someone be willing to allow others to improve?"*

Willingness—Responsibility

A1. *"What could you be responsible for?"*

A2. *"What could another be responsible for?"*

B1. *"What would be acceptable to be irresponsible about?"*

B2. *"What would be acceptable for another to be irresponsible about?"*

[*and then run*]

1. *"Spot a time when you made someone be responsible."*

2. *"Spot a time when someone made you be responsible."*

3. *"Spot a time when someone made another (or others) be responsible."*

[*and finally, run alternately (until the "glee" of "irresponsibility" is discharged)*]

A. *"Get a sense of the joy of responsibility."*

B. *"Get a sense of the joy of irresponsibility."*

DEFRAGMENTING "JUSTIFICATION"

For most of our participation in *Shared-Game Universes*, *Alpha-Spirits* have been operating from a point of *fragmentation*.

There is a mistaken, albeit *implanted,* "idea" or "goal" that we must be in *competition* with one another—that *"there can be only one"* or *"only one will survive."* There is, of course, no *actual* truth to this.

In order to reclaim the memory and abilities of our "past," it is necessary to be able to *confront* our actions (and the actions of others) in the "past" without *regret,* without *withdrawing* from the *imprints,* and without resorting to *justification* and *falsehood* (*altering* them) in order to make them more manageable. In *systematic processing,* we take some of the pressure off a *Seeker* by alternating PCL with *spotting* more positive things.

Domination—General

A. *"How have you dominated others?"*

B. *"Spot a way to enhance others."*

Domination—Stopping

A. *"How have you stopped others?"*

B. *"Spot a way to help others excel."*

Domination—Inhibition

A. *"How have you inhibited the survival of others?"*

B. *"Spot a way to aid the survival of others."*

"Domination" and *"Superiority"* are not the only *games* available to *Alpha-Spirits*. There are *better games* at higher levels of existence. However, in *this* present version of a *Physical Universe ("Beta-Existence")*—where physical *energy* and *force* are quite solid and supreme—these *games* are inherently the most common.

The type of "artificial" *fragmentation* that is *"implanted"* as *reality-agreements* for this *Universe*, instills a certain pattern of *"roles"* and *"goals"* for *this* particular *game*. This means that *all* of us have *something* that we use in order to gain our *"superiority"* over others—and we refer to this as a *"justification consideration."*

This primary *"justification consideration"* will be some basic characteristic that we

emphasize in exclusion to other things—so it *should* be easy to *recognize*. The *consideration* that we are after is also quite basic in structure. It will be a *basic goal*, such as: "to be holy" or "being intelligent" or "to be strong," *&tc.* Whatever it is, it is treated in *processing* as an "item" used to make yourself "*superior*" to others.

It takes this far along the *Pathway*—the amount of *Actualized Awareness* gained by this point of *systematic processing*—in order to *confront* such a *consideration* "*As-It-Is.*" The average *Human* will quickly *withdraw* from handling such things. But even the most "*Enlightened*" among us will still have this "*item*" on their "*track*"—the key difference being that they may have risen above the tendency to use it *against* others.

Although a more complete understanding of *games, goals* and the *Universes* representing them, is generally earned in the

most *upper-levels* of *Systemology*, it may be easily stated here that: employing your best characteristics in the low-grade *games* of *force* and *superiority* is quite "*unenlightened*." It causes a gradual deterioration of *abilities* and abandonment of a *goal* because of the *Harmful-Acts* that are required to maintain that specific type (or "*personality-role*") of "*superiority*" and "*rightness*" for "*dominance*."

Identifying and *recognizing* this primary "*justification consideration*" is not only necessary for completing *Systemology Level-3*, but is also the critical "*Key*" that "unlocks" (what we refer to as) the "*Backtrack*" for *upper-level processing* and additional "passes" through the *Professional Course* material.

The *game* of "*goals*" and "*roles*" extends back many "lifetimes" and many *Universes*. There is even an observable "systematic pattern" behind the way one *personality-type* and/or *goal* is abandoned,

requiring the individual to shift over to another that has not already deteriorated. So this particular "item" we are looking for is likely to be the same for a certain amount of former "lifetime" experiences, but not necessarily many (relatively speaking, compared to the larger scope of things).

For achieving a basic state of "*Beta-Defragmentation*," we primarily emphasize *this* lifetime. But, there are higher applications of this same *Professional Course* after it is completed once—such as additional "*Alpha-Defragmentation*" of the *Backtrack*. For present purposes, however, it is important to prefix certain PCL (such as our "search and discovery" of the primary "*justification consideration*") with "*In this lifetime...*" Later on, a *Seeker* can explore the *Backtrack* further.

It is important to approach this final area of *Systemology Level-3* with care, because accuracy is the only way to effectively

gain any stable progress from it. A *Seeker* should be in a state of high *Awareness* (having achieved "good" results from all former *processing*), be well rested (and alert), free of any actively *restimulative* sources of *fragmentation*, and finally, *interested* and *willing* to actually "discover" the "answer."

For this exercise, *list* your "answers" clearly. It's important not to do this while tired, because if you suddenly feel "heavy" or "tired" while *listing*, then you know you have *listed* too many answers —and that the basic answer you're looking for is already on the *list*. If after *listing* for a while, you start to feel "irritated" or "restimulated," then you still haven't put the answer you're looking for on the *list* yet.

Although this is a *listing exercise*, your *list* is not intended to be very long—in fact, you may *realize* what the answer is quite quickly. But, the basic instruction is to *list*

"answers" in your *notebook* (or *flight-log*) below where you have written out the "question" (PCL). You continue to *list* until you feel you have *"The Answer"* or you feel comfortable that you have *listed* enough.

When you find *"The Answer,"* this exercise is complete. If you're unsure which it is among your *list*, then go through it and consider each one in turn. When one doesn't seem like it's the right answer, put an "X" next to it, so you don't have to keep considering it. If at any point while checking your *list*, you suddenly *recognize "The Answer,"* then you stop working with the *list*. And, of course, if the *list* seems incomplete, you can always add to your *listed* answers until you've completed the exercise.

The *"Question"* (PCL) is:

"In this lifetime, what makes you superior to others?"

Then, when you have *"The Answer,"* write it in capital letters in your *notebook* (or *log*) and underline it. Take that "item" and use it to complete the next *process*. *Run* the following three PCL in alternation.

A. *"How does --- make you superior?"*

B. *"How could you use it to make yourself right?"*

C. *"How could you use it to make others wrong?"*

On the other side: we also want to find out what it is about others that you are (or might be) using against them. This might or might not relate to the *"roles"* and *"goals"* attached to the previously discovered *"justification consideration."* To find out, a *Seeker* performs another *listing exercise* (using the same basic instructions as before). This time, the PCL-*question* is:

"In this lifetime, what is it about others that makes them so wrong?"

If you aren't satisfied with the resulting answers, there is another way of using *processing*-PCL for a "search and discovery" (related to the previous exercise) which is:

"In this lifetime, what do you use to make others wrong?"

All of the exercises/*processes* in this section focus on finding out a *Seeker's "justification consideration"* (which is also tied to the *"roles"* and *"goals"* they are playing at in this lifetime). What it generally comes down to is a *basic consideration* that "others are evil," "others are stupid," or "they're weak," *&tc.* [These examples would respectively apply to *goals/roles* of "being good," "being intelligent," and "being strong."]

To *defragment* the *"justification consideration,"* we want to systematically untangle the *"negative"* associations of using our abilities against others, while still retain-

ing the original skill ("intelligence" or "strength," *&tc*).

The following *processes* are not *run* as simple alternating PCL. A *Seeker runs* a single PCL for as long as it continues to produce answers, then shifts to the second to get as many answers for that one, and then shifts back to the first PCL, and so on until the influential "intensity" of the *consideration* is dispersed (falls away).

Justification Consideration—
Right/Wrong

A. "*Spot ways that --- would make you right.*"

B. "*Spot ways that --- would make others wrong.*"

Justification Consideration—Domination

A. "*Spot ways that --- would help you escape domination.*"

B. "*Spot ways that --- would help you dominate others.*"

Justification Consideration — Survival

A. *"Spot ways that --- would aid your survival."*

B. *"Spot ways that --- would hinder the survival of others."*

The influential "intensity" that we speak of is the sense that the *consideration* is "true." When it is first treated in *processing*, the *consideration* may actually seem very much like the "truth" about "why people are the way they are" — and a *justification* for "why we are the way we are." By *spotting* this *consideration* with high-level *Awareness*, the "*charge*" behind the idea or concept (as being "true") starts to dissipate or disperse. A *Seeker* then *realizes* that this is a falsely held "belief" that keeps them from *Self-Honesty*.

Assisting or "helping" others improve in the same area as your "*justification consideration*" is one way that this *defragmentation* is maintained even after *processing*

sessions. It also helps to keep the *"goals"* and *"skills"* themselves from "deteriorating." For example: if your *goal* is "to be strong" (or a *role* of "being strong") and you viewed others as "wrong" for being "weak," the solution is to help others become "stronger," *&tc.*

This area is a very critical area for rehabilitation of other spiritual abilities and for rising above the limitations inherent in the standard-issue *Human Condition.* Therefore, a *Seeker* should not pass by this "checkpoint" on the *Pathway* without making certain that the *"justification consideration"* is properly found and *defragmented.* Such completes a *Seeker's processing* for *Systemology Level-3.*

The Systemology Professional Course
continues in the next lesson booklet:
CONFRONTING THE PAST

GLOSSARY

actualization : to make actual, not just potential; to bring into full solid Reality; to realize fully in *Awareness* as a "thing."

agreement (reality) : unanimity of opinion of what is "thought" to be known; an accepted arrangement of how things are; things we consider as "real" or as an "is" of "reality"; a consensus of what is real as made by standard-issue (common) participants; what an individual contributes to or accepts as "real"; in *Systemology*, a synonym for *"reality."*

alpha : the first, primary, basic, superior or beginning of some form; in *Systemology*, referring to the state of existence operating on spiritual archetypes and postulates, will and intention "exterior" to the low-level condensation and solidarity of energy and matter as the 'physical universe' (*beta*).

alpha-spirit : a "spiritual" *Life*-form; the "true" *Self* or I-AM; the *individual*; the spiritual (*alpha*) *Self* that is animating the (*beta*) physical body or *"genetic vehicle"* using a continuous *Lifeline* of spiritual ("*ZU*") energy; an individu-

al spiritual (*alpha*) entity possessing no physical mass or measurable waveform (motion) in the Physical Universe as itself, so it animates the (*beta*) physical body or "*genetic vehicle*" as a catalyst to experience *Self*-determined causality in effect within the *Physical Universe*; a singular unit or point of *Spiritual Awareness* that is *Aware* that it is *Aware.*

alpha thought : the highest spiritual *Self-determination* over creation and existence exercised by an Alpha-Spirit; the Alpha range of pure *Creative Ability* based on direct postulates and considerations of *Beingness*; spiritual qualities comparable to "thought" but originating in Alpha-existence, independently superior to a Mind-System.

ascension : actualized *Awareness* elevated to the point of true "spiritual existence" exterior to *beta existence.* An "Ascended Master" is one who has returned to an incarnation on Earth as an inherently *Enlightened One*, demonstrable in their words and actions; they have the ability to *Self-direct* the "Mind" and "Body" as *Self* (as a "Spirit"); and to maintain consciousness as a personal identity continuum with the same *Self-directed* control and communication of Will-Intention that is exercised, actualized and developed deliberately during one's present incarnation.

associative knowledge : significance or meaning of a facet or aspect assigned to (or considered to have) a direct relationship with another facet; to connect or relate ideas or facets of existence with one another; in traditional systems logic, an equivalency of significance or meaning between facets or sets that are grouped together, such as in *(a + b) + c = a + (b + c)*; in Systemology, erroneous associative knowledge is assignment of the same value to all facets or parts considered as related (even when they are not actually so), such as in *a = a, b = a, c = a* and so forth without distinction.

attention : active use of *Awareness* toward a specific aspect or thing; the act of "attending" with the presence of *Self*; a direction of focus or concentration of *Awareness* along a particular channel or conduit or toward a particular terminal node or communication termination point; the Self-directed concentration of personal energy as a combination of observation, thought-waves and consideration; focused application of *Self-Directed Awareness*.

awareness : the highest sense of-and-as *Self* in knowing and being as I-AM (the *Alpha-Spirit*); the extent of beingness directed as a viewpoint (POV) experienced by *Self* as *Knowingness*.

beta (existence) : all manifestation in the "Physical Universe" (KI, in *Zuism*); the conditions of *Awareness* for the *Alpha-spirit* (*Self*) as a physical organic *Lifeform* or "*genetic vehicle*" in which it experiences causality in the *Physical Universe*.

charge : to fill or furnish with a quality; to supply with energy; to lay a command upon; in *Systemology*—to imbue with intention; to overspread with emotion; personal energy stores and significances entwined as fragmentation in mental images, reactive-response encoding and intellectual (and/or) programmed beliefs.

circuit : a circular path or loop; a closed-path within a system that allows a flow; a pattern or action or wave movement that follows a specific route or potential path only; in *Systemology*, "*communication processing*" pertaining to a specific *flow* of energy or information along a channel; "*feedback loop.*"

communication : successful transmission of information, data, energy (&tc.) along a message line, with a reception of feedback; an energetic flow of intention to cause an effect (or duplication) at a distance; the personal energy moved or acted upon by will or else 'selective directed attention'; the 'messenger action' used to trans-

mit and receive energy across a medium; also relay of energy, a message or signal—or even locating a personal POV (viewpoint) for the Self—along the *ZU-line*.

confront : to come around in front of; to be in the presence of; to stand in front of, or in the face of; to meet "face-to-face" or "face-up-to"; additionally, in *Systemology*, to fully tolerate or acceptably withstand an encounter with a particular manifestation without an automatic reactive response..

consideration : careful analytical reflection of all aspects; deliberation; determining the significance of a "thing" in relation to similarity or dissimilarity to other "things"; evaluation of facts and importance of certain facts; thorough examination of all aspects related to, or important for, making a decision; the analysis of consequences and estimation of significance when making decisions; also in *Systemology*, the *postulate* or *Alpha-Thought* that defines the state of *beingness* for what something "*is*."

defragmentation : the *reparation* of wholeness; collecting all dispersed parts to reform an original whole; a process of removing "*fragmentation*" in data or knowledge to provide a clear understanding; applying techniques and processes that promote a *holistic* interconnected *al-*

pha state, favoring observational *Awareness* of continuity in all spiritual and physical systems; in *Systemology*, a "*Seeker*" achieving actualized "*Self-Honest Awareness*" is said to be in a basic state of *beta-defragmentation*, whereas *Alpha-defragmentation* is the rehabilitation of the *creative ability*, managing the *Spiritual Timeline* and the POV of *Self* as Alpha-Spirit (I-AM).

fragmentation : breaking into parts and scattering the pieces; the *fractioning* of wholeness or the *fracture* of a holistic interconnected *alpha* state, favoring observational *Awareness* of perceived connectivity between parts; *discontinuity*; separation of a totality into parts; in *Systemology*, a person outside of *Self-Honesty* is said to be operating from a *fragmented* state.

flow : movement across (or through) a channel (or conduit); a direction of active energetic motion, typically distinguished as either an *in-flow*, *out-flow* or *cross-flow*.

genetic-vehicle : a physical *Life*-form; the physical (*beta*) body that is animated/controlled by the (*Alpha*) *Spirit* using a continuous *Spiritual Lifeline* (ZU); a physical (*beta*) organic receptacle and catalyst for the (*Alpha*) *Self* to operate "causes" and experience "effects" within the *Physical Universe*.

harmful-act : a counter-survival mode of beha-

vior or action (esp. that causes harm to one of more *Spheres of Existence*)—or—an overtly aggressive (hostile and/or destructive) action against an individual or any other *Sphere of Existence*; in *Utilitarian Systemology*—a short-sighted (serves fewest/lowest *Spheres of Existence*) intentional overtly harmful action to resolve a perceived problem; a revision of the rule for standard *Utilitarianism* for Systemology to distinguish actions which provide the least benefit to the least number of *Spheres of Existence*, or else the greatest harm to the greatest number of *Spheres of Existence*; in *moral philosophy*—an action which can be experienced by few and/or which one would not be willing to experience for themselves (*theft, slander, rape, &tc*); an iniquity or iniquitous act.

hold-back : withheld communications (esp. actions) such as "*Hold-Outs*"; intentional (or automatic) withdrawal (as opposed to reach); Self-restraint (which may eventually be enforced or automated); not reaching, acting or expressing, when one should be; an ability that is now restrained (on automatic) due to inability to withhold it on Self-determinism alone.

hold-outs : in photography, the numerous snapshots/pictures withheld from the final display or

professional presentation of the event; withheld communications; in Utilitarian Systemology—energetic withdrawal and communication breaks with a "*terminal*" and its *Sphere of Existence* as a result of a "*Harmful-Act*"; unspoken or undiscovered (hidden, covert) actions that an individual withholds communications of, fearing punishment or endangerment of *Self-preservation* (*First Sphere*); the act of hiding (or keeping hidden) the truth of a "*Harmful-Act*"; a refusal to communicate with a *Pilot*; also "*Hold-Back.*"

holistic : the examination of interconnected systems as encompassing something greater than the *sum* of their "parts."

Human Condition : a standard default state of Human experience that is generally accepted to be the extent of its potential identity (*beingness*) —currently treated as *Homo Sapiens Sapiens,* but which is scheduled for replacement by *Homo Novus* (the "New Human").

imprint : to strongly impress, stamp, mark (or outline) onto a softer 'impressible' substance; to mark with pressure onto a surface; in *Systemology,* used to indicate permanent Reality impressions marked by frequencies, energies or interactions experienced during periods of emotional distress, pain, unconsciousness, loss, enforcement, or something antagonistic to

physical (personal) survival, all of which are are
stored with other reactive response-mechanisms
at lower-levels of *Awareness* as opposed to the
active memory database and proactive processing center of the Mind; an experiential
"memory-set" that may later resurface—be
triggered or stimulated artificially—as Reality,
of which similar responses will be engaged
automatically; holographic-like imagery
"stamped" onto consciousness as composed of
energetic *facets* tied to the "snap-shot" of an experience.

invalidate : decrease the level or degree or
agreement as Reality.

pilot : a professional steersman responsible for
healthy functional operation of a ship toward a
specific destination; in *Systemology*, an intensive trained individual qualified to specially apply *Systemology Processing* to assist other
Seekers on the *Pathway*.

point-of-view (POV) : a point to view from; an
opinion or attitude as expressed from a specific
identity-phase; a specific standpoint or vantage-
point; a definitive manner of consideration specific to an individual phase or identity; a place
or position affording a specific view or vantage;
circumstances and programming of an individual that is conducive to a particular response,

consideration or belief-set (paradigm); a position (consideration) or place (location) that provides a specific view or perspective (subjective) on experience (of the objective).

postulate : to put forward as truth; to suggest or assume an existence *to be*; to state or affirm the existence of particular conditions; to provide a basis of reasoning and belief; a basic theory accepted as fact; in *Systemology*, Alpha-Thought —the top-most decisions or considerations made by the Alpha-Spirit regarding the "*is-ness*" (what things "are") about energy-matter and space-time.

presence : a quality of some thing (*energy/matter*) being "present" in space-time; personal orientation of *Self* as an *Awareness* (*POV*) located in present space-time (environment) and communicating with extant energy-matter.

processing command line (PCL) or **command line** : a directed input; a specific command using highly selective language for *Systemology Processing*; a predetermined directive statement (cause) intended to focus concentrated attention (effect).

processing, systematic : the inner-workings or "through-put" result of systems; in *Systemology*, a method of applied spiritual technology used

toward personal Self-Actualization; methods of selective directed attention, communicated language and associative imagery that increases personal control of the human condition.

realization : the clear perception of an understanding; a consideration or understanding on what is "actual"; to make "real" or give "reality" to so as to grant a property of "beingness" or "being as it is"; the state or instance of coming to an *Awareness*; in *Systemology*, "gnosis" or true knowledge achieved during *systematic processing*; achievement of a new (or higher) cognition, true knowledge or perception of Self; a consideration of reality or assignment of meaning.

responsibility : the *ability* to *respond*; the extent of mobilizing *power* and *understanding* an individual maintains as *Awareness* to enact *change*; the proactive ability to *Self-direct* and make decisions independent of an outside authority.

Seeker : an individual on the *Pathway to Self-Honesty*; a practitioner of *Mardukite Systemology* or *Systemology Processing*, that is working toward *Spiritual Ascension*.

Self-actualization : bringing the full potential of the Human spirit into Reality; expressing full capabilities and creativeness of the *Alpha-Spirit*.

Self-determinism : the freedom to act, clear of external control or influence; the personal control of Will to direct intention.

Self-honesty : the basic or original *alpha* state of *being* and *knowing*; clear and present total *Awareness* of-and-as *Self*, in its most basic and true proactive expression of itself as *Spirit* or *I-AM*—free of artificial attachments, perceptive filters and other emotionally-reactive or mentally-conditioned programming imposed on the human condition by the systematized physical world; the ability to experience existence without judgment.

spiritual timeline : a continuous stream of moment-to-moment *Mental Images* (or a record of experiences) that defines the "past" of a spiritual being (or *Alpha-Spirit*) and which includes impressions (*imprints, &tc.*) from all life-incarnations and significant spiritual events the being has encountered; in Systemology, also "*backtrack.*"

Spheres of Existence : a series of *eight* concentric circles, rings or spheres (each larger than the former) that is overlaid onto the Standard Model of Beta-Existence to demonstrate the dynamic systems of existence extending out from the POV of Self (often as a "body") at the *First Sphere*; these are given in the basic eightfold

systems as: *Self, Home/Family, Groups, Humanity, Life on Earth, Physical Universe, Spiritual Universe* and *Infinity-Divinity*.

Systemology : a modern tradition of applied religious philosophy and spiritual technology based on *Arcane Tablets* (in combination with "*general systemology*" and "*games theory*") developed in the New Age underground by Joshua Free in 2011 as an advanced futurist extension of the *Mardukite Research Org.*; also known as "*Mardukite Systemology,*" "*Metahuman Systemology*" and "*Spiritual Systemology.*"

terminal (node) : a point, end, or mass, on a line; a connection point for closing an electric circuit, such as a post on a battery terminating at each end of its own systematic function; a point of connectivity with other points; in systems, a contact point of interaction; a point of interaction with other points.

turbulence : a quality or state of distortion or disturbance that creates irregularity of a flow or pattern; the quality or state of aberration on a line (such as ragged edges) or the emotional "turbulent feelings" attached to a particular flow or terminal node; a violent, haphazard or disharmonious commotion (such as in the ebb of gusts and lulls of wind action).

validation : a reinforcement of agreements or considerations as being "real."

viewpoint : see "*point-of-view" (POV).*

willingness : the state of conscious Self-determined ability and interest (directed attention) to *Be*, *Do* or *Have*; a Self-determined consideration to reach, face up to (*confront*) or manage some "mass" or energy; the extent to which an individual considers themselves able to participate, act or communicate along some line, to put attention or intention on the line, or to produce (create) an effect.

ZU : the ancient Sumerian cuneiform sign for the archaic verb—"*to know*," "*knowingness*" or "*awareness*"; in *Mardukite Zuism and Systemology*, the active energy/matter of the "Spiritual Universe" (AN) experienced as a *Lifeforce* or *consciousness* that imbues living forms extant in the "Physical Universe" (KI); "*Spiritual Life Energy*"; energy demonstrated by the WILL of an actualized *Alpha-Spirit* in the "Spiritual Universe" (AN), which impinges its *Awareness* into the Physical Universe (KI), animating/controlling *Life* for its experience of *beta-existence* along an individual Alpha-Spirit's personal *Identity-continuum*, called a *ZU-line*.

Zu-**Line** : a theoretical construct in *Mardukite*

Zuism and Systemology demonstrating *Spiritual Life Energy* (*ZU*) as a personal individual "continuum" of Awareness interacting with all Spheres of Existence on the Standard Model of Systemology; a spectrum of potential variations and interactions of a monistic continuum or singular *Spiritual Life Energy* demonstrated on the Standard Model; an energetic channel of potential POV and "locations" of Beingness, demonstrated in early Systemology materials as an individual Alpha-Spirit's personal *Identity- continuum*, potentially connecting *Awareness* of *Self* with "*Infinity*" simultaneous with all points considered in existence; a symbolic demonstration of the "*Life-line*" on which *Awareness (ZU)* extends from the direction of the "Spiritual Universe" (AN) in its true original *alpha state* through an entire possible range of activity resulting in its *beta state* and control of a *genetic-entity* occupying the *Physical Universe (KI)*.

Zu-Vision : the true and basic (*Alpha*) Point-of-View (perspective, POV) maintained by *Self* as *Alpha-Spirit* outside boundaries or considerations of the *Human Condition* and *exterior* to beta-existence reality agreements with the Physical Universe; a POV of Self *as* "a unit of Spiritual Awareness" that exists independent of a "body" and entrapment in a *Human Condition*; "spirit vision" in its truest sense.

Fundamentals of Systemology
in six
Basic Course Lesson Booklets

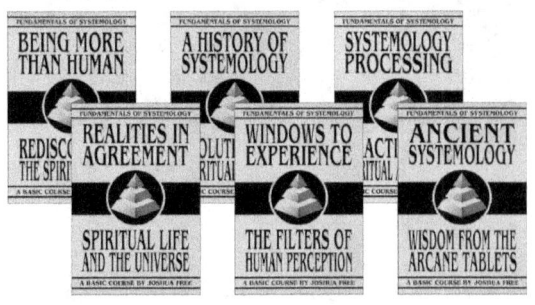

Also
available
as a
six-in-one
hardcover
edition!

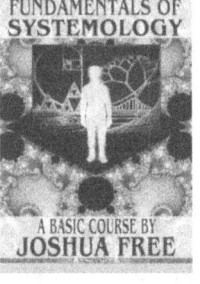

THE SYSTEMOL

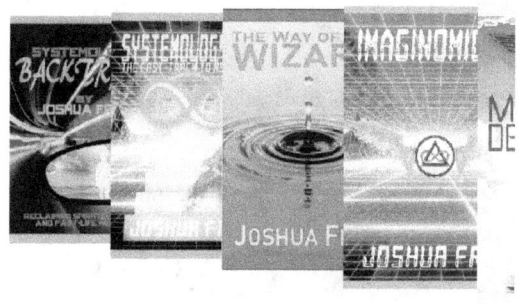

Seekers and students of the *Basic Course* and *Professional Course* will also be interested in the *Advanced Series* of the *Systemology Core.* These volumes are a complete chronological record of the Mardukite New Thought developments from the Systemology Society, published in 2019 through 2023.

The *Systemology Core* begins with the first professional publication released when the *Mardukite Systemology Society* emerged from the underground in 2019, with: *"The Tablets of Destiny Revelation."*

OGY PATHWAY

The Tablets of Destiny Revelation:
*How Long-Lost Anunnaki Wisdom
Can Change the Fate of Humanity*

Crystal Clear: *Handbook for Seekers*

Metahuman Destinations (2 *volumes*)

Imaginomicon:
Approaching Gateways to Higher Universes

Way of the Wizard: *Utilitarian Systemology*

Systemology-180: *Fast-Track to Ascension*

Systemology Backtrack:
Reclaiming Spiritual Power & Past-Life Memory

PUBLISHED BY THE **JOSHUA FREE** IMPRINT REPRESENTING

The Mardukite Academy of Systemology

THE JOSHUA FREE IMPRINT
JFI PUBLICATIONS

MARDUKITE
ZUISM

mardukite.com

www.ingramcontent.com/pod-product-compliance
Lightning Source LLC
Chambersburg PA
CBHW071212120626
46546CB00006B/2526